T0073396

Appalachian Health

APPALACHIAN HEALTH

Culture, Challenges, and Capacity

Edited by F. Douglas Scutchfield and
Randy Wykoff

Foreword by Alonzo Plough

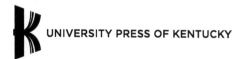

UNIVERSITY PRESS OF KENTUCKY

Scholarly publisher for the Commonwealth,
serving Bellarmine University, Berea College, Centre
College of Kentucky, Eastern Kentucky University,
The Filson Historical Society, Georgetown College,
Kentucky Historical Society, Kentucky State University,
Morehead State University, Murray State University,
Northern Kentucky University, Spalding University,
Transylvania University, University of Kentucky,
University of Louisville, and Western Kentucky University.
All rights reserved.

Editorial and Sales Offices: The University Press of Kentucky
663 South Limestone Street, Lexington, Kentucky 40508-4008
www.kentuckypress.com

Library of Congress Cataloging-in-Publication Data

Names: Scutchfield, F. Douglas, editor. | Wykoff, Randolph, editor.
Title: Appalachian health : culture, challenges, and capacity / edited by
    F. Douglas Scutchfield and Randy Wykoff ; foreword by Alonzo Plough
Description: Lexington, Kentucky : The University Press of Kentucky, [2022] |
    Includes bibliographical references and index.
Identifiers: LCCN 2021039336 | ISBN 9780813155579 (hardcover ; alk. paper) |
    ISBN 9780813155883 (pdf) | ISBN 9780813155937 (epub)
Subjects: MESH: Medically Underserved Area | Health Services Accessibility |
    Socioeconomic Factors | Appalachian Region
Classification: LCC RA566.4.A66 | NLM W 76 AA6 | DDC 362.109756/8—dc23

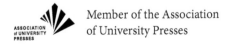

Member of the Association
of University Presses

Contents

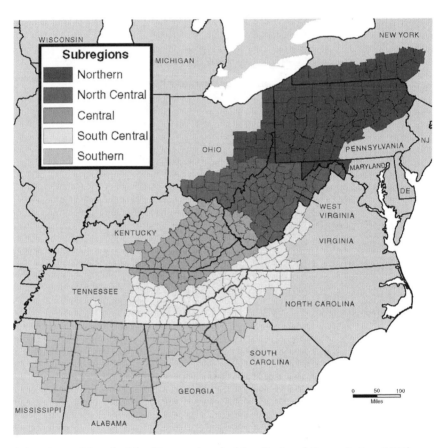

Subregions of Appalachia. (*Source:* Appalachian Regional Commission, 2009)

Foreword

Appalachia is often discussed in statistical abstractions or characterized by researchers without lived experience in the region. This book's editors and contributors offer a wonderful and timely correction to this pattern, as their voices are informed by deep knowledge of the places, the history, and the context of Appalachia.

This framing makes explicit the social, political, economic, and environmental conditions and forces that ultimately determine health and well-being anywhere. The chapters combine excellent research summaries and data analysis with a nuanced presentation of the changing economic context and shifts in the region's traditional industries, such as coal. The contributors balance data and storytelling to capture the subtleties of a region encompassing parts of thirteen very different states.

The authors employ an analytic framework based on the broad social determinants of health. This framework allows them to integrate discussions of the myriad challenges influencing the health of the people of Appalachia. For instance, access to affordable and timely medical care is connected to the geographic barriers in this mountainous and largely rural region. The environmental toxins that cause a high prevalence of specific diseases such as COPD in the region are connected to the problematic legacy of coal mining. The declining economic vitality of the coal industry itself has contributed to the growing poverty and marginalization of many residents of Appalachia. These economic conditions contribute to the despair and hopelessness that can lead to medical problems such as opioid addiction. The authors weave and connect these seemingly separate issues in a way that allows a better understanding of the past and points to the possibility of a brighter future for the region.

Readers of this book will see that improving the health and well-being of the Appalachian people has always been rooted in the enduring strength of the region's individuals and culture. However, this strength must be augmented by local, state, and federal policies that support economic revitalization and investment in schools and health care capacity. Change must be driven by community voices and the life experiences of the Appalachian people through processes that build trust in systems and leaders. There are communities in the region where this process is happening right now. At the Robert Wood Johnson Foundation, we call this building a culture of health that gives everyone a fair and just opportunity to achieve the best possible health and well-being. Like the authors of this book, we see hope and promise for improved health in Appalachia.

Alonzo Plough
Chief Science Officer and Vice President
Robert Wood Johnson Foundation

Abbreviations

ACA	Patient Protection and Affordable Care Act of 2010
AHRQ	Agency for Healthcare Research and Quality
ANOVA	analysis of variance
AP	advanced placement
APRN	advance practice registered nurse
ARC	Appalachian Regional Commission
ARDA	Appalachian Regional Development Act of 1965
ARH	Appalachian Regional Hospitals (now Healthcare)
ASA	Appalachian Studies Association
ASD	Appalachian Sustainable Development
ASPE	assistant secretary for planning and evaluation
BMI	body mass index
BRFSS	Behavioral Risk Factor Surveillance System
BTU	British thermal unit
CAH	critical access hospital
CARES	Coronavirus Aid, Relief, and Economic Security Act of 2020
CCP	Correctional Career Pathways (program)
CDC	Centers for Disease Control and Prevention
CHC	community health center
CHW	community health worker
CLAS	culturally and linguistically appropriate services
CMS	Centers for Medicare & Medicaid Services
CNM	certified nurse midwife (APRN with additional certification)
COPD	chronic obstructive pulmonary disease
CPSTF	Community Preventive Service Task Force
CSHIB	US Chemical Safety and Hazard Investigation Board
DEA	Drug Enforcement Administration
DHHS	US Department of Health and Human Services
DHP	demonstration health project
EPA	Environmental Protection Agency
ERS	Economic Research Service (of the USDA)
ESRI	Environmental Systems Research Institute
ETSU	East Tennessee State University
FBI	Federal Bureau of Investigation

FEMA	Federal Emergency Management Agency
FFL	Fit for Life (program)
FNS	Frontier Nursing Service
FNU	Frontier Nursing University
FQHC	federally qualified health center
GDP	gross domestic product
HEAL	Helping to End Addiction Long-term (initiative)
HEPPA	Health Education for Prenatal Providers in Appalachia
HINTS	Health Information National Trends Survey
HPV	human papillomavirus
IOM	Institute of Medicine
KH	Kentucky Homeplace
MCHM	4-methlycyclohexanemethanol
MMHA	Miners Memorial Hospital Association
MOUD	medication for opioid use disorder
MSHA	Mine Safety and Health Administration
NAFTA	North American Free Trade Agreement
NCCDCPHP	National Center for Chronic Disease Control and Prevention and Health Promotion
NCHS	National Center for Health Statistics
NCI	National Cancer Institute
NHSC	National Health Service Corps
NIH	National Institutes of Health
NORC	NORC at the University of Chicago
NP	nurse practitioner
NVSS	National Vital Statistics System
OB-GYN	obstetrician-gynecologist
OECD	Organisation for Economic Co-operation and Development
OPR	opioid pain reliever
OUD	opioid use disorder
PA	physician assistant
PARC	President's Appalachian Regional Commission (ARC's predecessor)
PCP	primary care provider (or physician)
PDMP	prescription drug monitoring program
PED	pediatrician
PHEP	Public Health Emergency Preparedness (program)
PIU	Plate It Up
POE	Proactive Office Encounter
RHIhub	Rural Health Information Hub

RTIP	Research-Tested Intervention Program
RWJF	Robert Wood Johnson Foundation
SAMHSA	Substance Abuse and Mental Health Services Administration
SDOH	social determinants of health
SIDS	sudden infant death syndrome
SLRP	State Loan Repayment Program
SMCRA	Surface Mining Control and Reclamation Act of 1977
SSB	sugar-sweetened beverage
SSP	syringe services program
SUD	substance use disorder
SWV	Southern West Virginia
TFAH	Trust for America's Health
TNIPH	Tennessee Institute of Public Health
tPA	tissue plasminogen activator
TVA	Tennessee Valley Authority
UIC	urban influence code
UMWA	United Mine Workers of America
USDA	US Department of Agriculture
USEIA	US Energy Information Administration
WHO	World Health Organization
WRF	Welfare and Retirement Fund (of UMWA)
YPLL	years of potential life lost
YRBSS	Youth Risk Behavior Surveillance System

1

Introduction

F. Douglas Scutchfield and Randy Wykoff

> I shall not leave these prisoning hills
> Though they topple their barren heads to level earth
> And the forests slide uprooted out of the sky.
> Though the waters of Troublesome, of Trace Fork,
> Of Sand Lick rise in a single body to glean the valleys,
> To drown lush pennyroyal, to unravel rail fences;
> Though the sun-ball breaks the ridges into dust
> And burns its strength into the blistered rock
> I cannot leave. I cannot go away.
>
> Being of these hills, being one with the fox
> Stealing into the shadows, one with the new-born foal,
> The lumbering ox drawing green beech logs to mill,
> One with the destined feet of man climbing and descending,
> And one with death rising to bloom again, I cannot go.
> Being of these hills I cannot pass beyond.
>
> *James Still, "Heritage"*

Why Appalachia?

This book is about the health and well-being of the people of Appalachia and the many social, economic, geographic, and medical factors that have long distinguished the region from the rest of the United States. Why study the people of Appalachia? In many ways, this is both a simple and a complex question. It is simple because the people of Appalachia, and the residents of other rural and isolated parts of the country, are currently in the national consciousness. Appalachia is, in many ways, an economic and political bellwether for the United States. Periodically, the national political discourse prompts the media to refocus their attention on the problems and issues of the people of Appalachia, after these issues have been out of the public eye for some time. One of the best examples is the iconic picture of Lyndon Johnson "hunkered down" (as the mountain folks say) to talk about jobs on the porch of an unemployed mill worker in Martin County, Kentucky (figure 1.1). Johnson used this

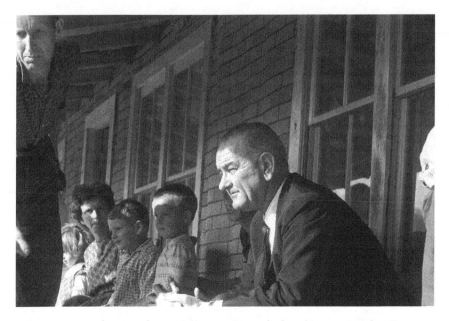

Figure 1.1. President Lyndon B. Johnson in Appalachia. (*Source:* Lyndon B. Johnson Library Archive; photograph by Cecil Stoughton)

photo opportunity as a prelude to announcing his War on Poverty in 1964. Others have used Appalachia either to highlight a presidential initiative or to campaign for the office. Both John F. Kennedy and Robert Kennedy visited the mountains while running for the presidency, as did Bill Clinton.

During these times of national attention, the well-being of the people of Appalachia becomes part of the national dialogue, and they are viewed sympathetically as an example of the challenges facing the country. However, the 2016 presidential election may have changed this sympathetic view of the Appalachian people. In that election, the majority of the region's voters, despite their traditional affiliation with the Democratic Party, cast their ballots for the Republican candidate, Donald Trump. Indeed, the people of Appalachia (and voters in other economically depressed regions) were thought to be largely responsible for Trump's election. They have since been cast as his base: disaffected, disadvantaged, discouraged, and, in an economic sense, displaced.

This view is not entirely correct: Appalachia and other rural areas were not the sole source of President Trump's victory. In addition to carrying all but two of the states containing parts of Appalachia (the exceptions being New York and Virginia, where the Appalachian counties are a very small minority), Trump won most of the rest of the country, geographically speaking. Nevertheless, some people view Appalachians (and their counterparts in other rural areas) as the force that propelled Trump to the White House. This perceived political importance of Appalachia has once again motivated the rest of America—and especially the media—to reexamine the region in an attempt to understand the political dynamics there, as evidenced by the *New Yorker's* "In the Heart of Trump Country" and PBS's "Once a Clinton Stronghold, Appalachia Now Trump Country." Through these explorations, journalists have attempted to outline the myriad factors that caused the people of Appalachia to move away from their traditional party affiliation and seemingly to repudiate many of the social programs designed to help them.[1]

Thus, the simple answer to the question why study the people of Appalachia is that Appalachians are, once again, squarely in the public eye. The more complex answer—and the more important one—is that there are real and significant challenges (economic, social, medical, and others) that impact the health and well-being of the region's people. These factors are not, of course, unique to Appalachia; thus, understanding (and ultimately addressing) them could improve the welfare of Americans in all parts of the country, especially those who have not benefited from the nation's economic growth. For example, the decline of the coal industry, which has increased unemployment in major West Virginia, eastern Kentucky, and eastern Tennessee communities, is not fundamentally dissimilar to the decline of manufacturing in the Rust Belt or the decline of textiles in the Southeast. Certainly, over the coming century, many other sectors will evolve and change, placing entire regions on a downward economic trajectory. This type of decline is associated with many other challenges that will be marked, in region after region, by worsening health, social, and economic cycles.

Yet we can influence these trends if we systematically evaluate and understand similar processes in Appalachia. Doing this work requires clear acknowledgment of the fact that Appalachia is not monolithic, although the counties within the region do share marked health-related inequalities. In speaking of "the persistent poverty and human suffering in the mountains," Eller paints a picture of the region's complex landscape. He notes that "the decline of coal mining jobs due largely to changing markets; the absence of employment alternatives; the rise of opiate addiction; higher rates of depression, heart disease, and cancer; growing dependence upon Medicaid and SSI [supplemental security income]; and insufficient tax revenues for education and other local services continues to set Appalachia apart as one of the most distressed parts of rural America more than five decades after Lyndon Johnson declared his War on Poverty."[2]

Why Appalachian Health?

The first step in studying the health and well-being of the people of Appalachia is to analyze the interrelated cycles of social, economic, medical, and other conditions that have produced the region's current health status. The second step is to develop strategies that can interrupt these cycles—in Appalachia and elsewhere. Understanding the interrelationship among these factors will help guide the nation's response to future health challenges, wherever they occur.

Many Americans presume that their health is among the best in the world. However, although the United States spends substantially more on health and health care than any other developed nation, this investment has not translated into improved health status. In fact, the United States is one of the least healthy of the world's advanced economies. As 2018 data from the Organisation for Economic Co-operation and Development (OECD) show, despite the United States' outsized spending on health care, Americans' overall life expectancy trails that of the majority of economically developed countries (figure 1.2).[3]

According to the Institute of Medicine (IOM), which compared US health indicators to those in sixteen other "peer" countries in 2013, there are nine areas in which the United States lags behind:

- Adverse birth outcomes: The United States fares worse than many countries in infant mortality and low-birth-weight babies.
- Injuries and homicides: The United States outpaces its peers in vehicular and non-traffic-related injuries, as well as violent deaths.
- Adolescent pregnancy and sexually transmitted disease: Among developed nations, the United States has the highest rate of pregnant teenagers and sexually transmitted disease.
- HIV and AIDS: The United States is second among its peers in the prevalence of HIV infection, and it is number one in the incidence of AIDS.
- Drug-related mortality: More years of life are lost in the United States to alcohol and other drugs, even when drunk-driving deaths are excluded, than in any other peer nation.
- Obesity and diabetes: The United States is the most obese country among its peers, and it leads all others in the prevalence of diabetes among those older than twenty.
- Heart disease: The United States is second among developed nations in heart disease mortality prior to age fifty; Americans older than fifty are more likely to have cardiovascular disease and die of it than individuals in peer nations.

- Chronic lung disease: The United States is worse than all European countries in the prevalence of and mortality from lung disease.
- Disability: The United States has a higher rate of arthritis and activity limitation than European countries and Japan.

Though many of these health disparities exist across the economic spectrum, the vast majority are worse in Appalachia.[4]

The IOM report describes potential contributors to US health disparities, including a fragmented health care delivery system that is driven by volume, not value, and in which consumers must structure their own set of providers to receive the breadth of care required. It also cites the health habits and behaviors of Americans, who consume more calories, abuse more prescription drugs, use seatbelts less frequently, have more drunk-driving accidents, have easier access to firearms, and are more likely to become sexually active at an earlier age and have more sexual partners than individuals in other nations. Additionally, Americans have higher poverty rates (particularly among children) and a higher rate of income inequality, and the US government spends fewer funds on "safety net" programs. This last point is particularly important, as research has demonstrated that social spending in developed nations is inversely related to health outcomes. In other words, countries that spend money on education, food support, housing, transportation, employment, and social support enjoy a better health status. Finally, there is substantial evidence that the built environment can positively influence health status. For instance, many other developed nations are providing incentives for people to bicycle to work, thus encouraging physical activity while simultaneously decreasing mortality and morbidity associated with auto accidents and environmental pollution.[5]

As highlighted in this book, many of the same factors that cause health disparities between the United States and other countries result in the people of Appalachia being considerably less healthy than the rest of the nation. Braveman and colleagues note that health disparities are "systematic, plausibly avoidable health differences according to race or ethnicity, skin color, religion, or nationality; socioeconomic resources or position (reflected by, for example, income, wealth, education, or occupation); gender, sexual orientation, gender identity; age, geography, disability, illness, political or other affiliation; or other characteristics associated with discrimination or marginalization." Clearly, Appalachia is a region with substantial health disparities. Moreover, its large geographic size magnifies the importance of efforts like ours to understand the roots of poor health outcomes; Appalachia encompasses 428 counties and more than 25 million people, making up about 8 percent of the US population and accounting for a large proportion of its health, economic, and social challenges.

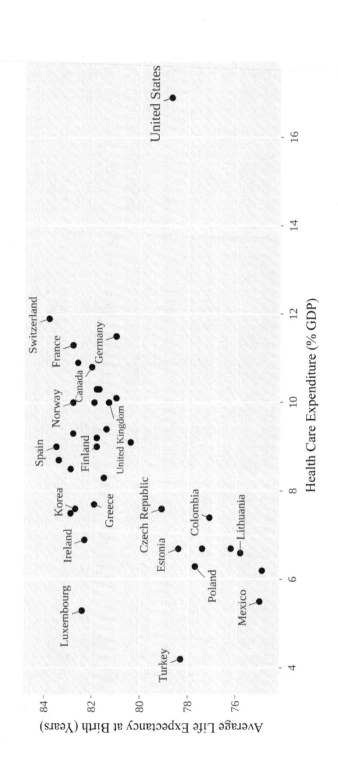

Figure 1.2. Life expectancy versus health care expenditures (percentage of gross domestic product) among OECD countries, 2018.

As reported by Egen and colleagues, extreme poverty in the United States is widely dispersed, with the poorest 2 percent of counties being located in thirteen different states. However, more than a quarter of those poorest counties are in Appalachia, making it an ideal region to study and gain a better understanding of the health challenges of all socially disadvantaged Americans.[6]

A pivotal study of disparities and inequities is that by Murray and colleagues, who examined life expectancies in race-county combinations in the United States. The study divided the United States into "eight Americas": Asian; northern low-income rural white (Northland); Middle America; Appalachian and lower Mississippi Valley low-income white (Appalachia); western Native American; black Middle America; southern low-income rural black; and high-risk urban black. They found that low-income whites in Appalachia with an average income similar to that of their counterparts in the Northland have a life expectancy equal to that of residents of Mexico and Panama and much lower than that of Americans in the Northland. In 2001 the life expectancy gap between whites in the Northland and in Appalachia was 4.2 and 3.8 years for males and females, respectively, compared with gaps of 6.4 and 4.6 years between whites and blacks as a whole. The gap between whites in the Northland and Appalachia had increased since 1982, when it was 3.0 and 2.4 years for males and females, respectively.[7]

Among the sources of data on the health status of the people of Appalachia is Health Disparities in Appalachia, an innovative research initiative sponsored by the Robert Wood Johnson Foundation (RWJF) and the Appalachian Regional Commission (ARC) and administered by the Foundation for a Healthy Kentucky. Thirty-three of the forty-one evaluated indicators are worse in Appalachia than in the rest of the country; these include both health factors (drug overdose, obesity, smoking, physical inactivity) and health outcomes (including seven of the ten leading causes of death: heart disease, cancer, chronic obstructive pulmonary disease, injury, stroke, diabetes, and suicide). Appalachia ranked better than the United States overall in only eight of the forty-one indicators: HIV prevalence, travel time to work, excessive drinking, student-teacher ratio, chlamydia prevalence, percentage of the population under age sixty-five that is uninsured, diabetes monitoring among Medicare patients, and social association rate. Appalachia also has fewer health care professionals when compared with the United States as a whole, including primary care physicians, mental health providers, specialty physicians, and dentists. Lower household incomes and higher poverty rates reflect worse living conditions in the region than in the nation as a whole.[8]

An analysis of county health rankings shows that, in the four states that make up Central Appalachia (Kentucky, West Virginia, Virginia, and Tennessee), there are dramatic differences between the 238 Appalachian counties and the 353 non-Appalachian counties. In all health outcome and health behavior metrics, the Appalachian counties perform worse than the non-Appalachian counties; in fact, the latter counties generally perform as well as, or better than, the national averages. These data clearly demonstrate that, as a whole, the 238 counties of Central Appalachia have significantly worse health statistics than the 2,903 US counties that are not in Central Appalachia and the 353 non-Appalachian counties within the Central Appalachian states. To demonstrate how marked this difference is within states, Woolf and colleagues examined Kentucky's life expectancy by county and found that it decreases steadily as one travels down the Mountain Parkway. In urban Fayette County (home to Lexington), life expectancy is seventy-eight years, while it is a mere seventy years in Wolfe County, a rural, impoverished Appalachian county.[9]

This long-standing and widespread inequity in Appalachia—a region in one of the richest countries in history—suggests why this unique group of Americans deserves our attention and our help in understanding and addressing the many causes of disparity. We hope that a study of the challenges facing the Appalachian people will help the nation better understand the challenges facing all rural people and, equally, all impoverished people, urban and rural alike.

Organization of the Book

Chapter 2 explores the health and well-being of the people of Appalachia by making an effort to understand the people themselves—their culture, their history, and the geographic region in which they live. Chapter 3 explores the health status of Appalachians living in the rest of the country. This sets the stage for an analysis of the factors that cause the identified health disparities. Subsequent chapters focus on the causal factors themselves, examining the behavioral, socioecological, environmental (broadly defined), and medical care determinants of health in this population and assessing the extent to which each of these factors distinguishes Appalachia from the rest of the country.

In this effort, we follow the model laid out by the County Health Rankings program of the University of Wisconsin, in conjunction with the RWJF (figure 1.3). This model emphasizes several points, most notably that health policy influences health factors, which in turn influence health outcomes, including the length and quality of life. This progression is clear in the example of anti-smoking laws, which affect tobacco use within a population and thereby influence mortality and morbidity associated with lung cancer, for example. The layperson generally believes that health disparities are due to a lack of access to

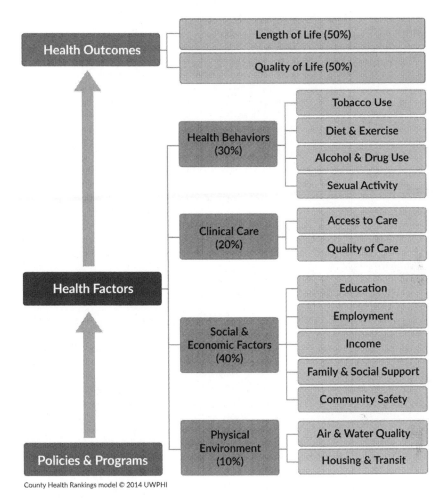

Figure 1.3. County Health Rankings model. (*Source:* University of Wisconsin Population Health Institute, 2016)

health care services, but this model suggests that medical care accounts for only 20 percent of the total contribution to health outcomes. According to this model, the two most important factors affecting health outcomes are social and economic factors (40 percent of the total) and health behaviors (30 percent). The health behaviors of concern in Appalachia include smoking, obesity, physical inactivity, and drug abuse.[10]

Chapter 4 turns to the socioeconomic factors that impact health in Appalachia. From the County Health Rankings model, it is apparent that these

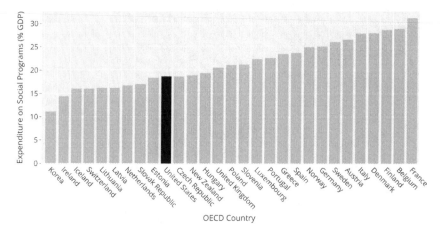

Figure 1.4. Spending on social programs (percentage of gross domestic product) among OECD countries, 2018.

Source: "Social Expenditure—Aggregated Data, 2018," *OECD*. Stat *Database* (October 20, 2020), https://stats.oecd.org/.

factors have the greatest influence on health. Their effect is especially marked in parts of the country that are experiencing socioecological problems. Problems such as poverty, lack of education, economic inequities, and job loss color many Appalachian communities. The interrelationship between health and these factors is becoming an increasingly important issue. Moreover, these factors are difficult to modify because they require a change in social policy—always a contentious undertaking—and involve the equally sensitive issue of capital inequality. The politicization of these issues makes it harder to justify using health funding to address socioeconomic determinants. However, there appears to be a relationship between spending on social programs and health, and the United States has not contributed to these programs as readily as other developed nations have (figure 1.4). Regardless of how difficult resource allocation is, it remains a key issue for those interested in improving health status.

Chapter 5 focuses on the occurrence of certain health behaviors in Appalachia and considers macrolevel approaches to modifying these behaviors. The drug abuse problem is affecting the entire nation, but it is having a major impact on Appalachia. This impact manifests not only in a rapidly increasing number of overdose deaths but also in co-occurring disorders—such as hepatitis C and HIV—and in the myriad economic factors accompanying drug-related crime, incarceration, and family disruption. Thus, drug abuse is discussed separately in chapter 9.

Chapter 6 examines the issues surrounding medical care and access to that care in Appalachia. Although health care is not primarily responsible for health outcomes, it receives the majority of attention and resources in Appalachia and beyond. For example, much of ARC's investment in health has been focused on the development of health services infrastructure rather than on socioecological factors, which are the major drivers of health status. The chapter first explores financial access to medical care. The Patient Protection and Affordable Care Act (ACA) has had a major impact on the region. This is particularly true in those states that have opted to use this mechanism to expand Medicaid coverage to all those in poverty. Then it examines the health assets of Appalachia resulting from infrastructure development, demonstrating that attention to systemic needs has resulted in some redress of the geographic barriers to access through community health centers, the Appalachia Regional Healthcare System, and some special programs and activities such as the Frontier Nursing Service. Finally, the chapter analyzes the supply of health care personnel, which has been a major issue in Appalachia. Many government resources have been expended to correct the geographic maldistribution of health care professionals. Major attention has been given to the availability of physicians in the region, but the maldistribution applies to other health care professionals as well.

Chapter 7 covers the environment: ambient, work, and built. Due to its historical ties to coal mining, Appalachia faces major work-related environmental issues and controversies. To illustrate, Appalachia has a high prevalence of occupational pulmonary diseases (both silicosis and anthracosis) as a result of miners' exposure to rock dust and coal dust. In addition, deep mining is associated with a substantial increase in musculoskeletal diseases (both acute and chronic). There is significant controversy over the extent to which mountaintop-removal mining results in an increased incidence of disease close to these mining sites.[11] The interpretation of the epidemiology data has led to "dueling epidemiologists"—those from the academy versus those hired by the coal industry. Also of concern is the built environment, which refers to the physical layout of communities, of what materials and how that environment is built, and the location of certain assets—for example, the occurrence of "food deserts," where there are no grocery stores to provide fresh fruits and vegetables year-round. In addition, many Appalachian communities—particularly smaller, more rural ones—lack sidewalks and bike trails and have other issues that make physical activity more difficult, contributing to sedentary lifestyles, obesity, and its sequel, diabetes.

Chapters 8 and 9 focus on specific issues in Appalachia that are of increasing concern. As noted earlier, chapter 9 addresses drug abuse, which has become a major concern with the rapid rise of opioid use. An associated issue is covered in chapter 8: so-called deaths of despair. Case and Deaton described this phenomenon in 2015 as a situation in which white, poorly educated, midlife Americans experience an increasing mortality rate associated with drug abuse, suicide, alcohol use, and chronic diseases such as cancer and heart disease. Subsequent work by Meit and colleagues found that this phenomenon exists among individuals from Appalachia.[12]

Chapter 10, on public health preparedness, highlights the unique challenges created by exogenous shocks in the region, such as flooding and the COVID-19 pandemic.

The conclusion of the book summarizes the relevant issues and problems and the potential means of addressing them. It includes the recommendation that the health of Appalachia's citizens be approached with sensitivity and care. Appalachia suffers from a substantial set of disparities in many areas, but most often they manifest as poor health status. Yet this need not be the case, as the region has many natural assets, including its people. How can we address these issues and create the structural changes needed to equalize the health status of Appalachia's people with that of other Americans? We hope this book goes a long way in providing an answer.

Notes

Epigraph: James Still, "Heritage," in *From the Mountain, from the Valley: New and Collected Poems* (Lexington: University Press of Kentucky, 2013), 43.

1. Larissa MacFarquar, "In the Heart of Trump Country," *New Yorker,* October 3, 2016, https://www.newyorker.com/magazine/2016/10/10/in-the-heart-of-trump-country; Lisa Lerer, "Once a Clinton Stronghold, Appalachia Now Trump Country," PBS, May 3, 2016, https://www.pbs.org/newshour/nation/once-a-clinton-stronghold-appalachia-now-trump-country.

2. Ron Eller, "Appalachia in the Age of Trump" (lecture, University of Kentucky Department of History, Lexington, September 28, 2017).

3. OECD, "Health Statistics," http://www.oecd.org/health/health-statistics.htm.

4. Institute of Medicine and National Research Council, *U.S. Health in International Perspective: Shorter Lives, Poorer Health* (Washington, DC: National Academies Press, 2013).

5. Megan Reynolds and Mauricio Avendano, "Social Policy Expenditure and Life Expectancy in High-Income Countries," *American Journal of Preventive Medicine* 54, no. 1 (2018): 72–79; Ryan E. Rhodes, Ian Janssen, Shannon S. D. Bredin, Darren E. R. Warburton, and Adrian Bauman, "Physical Activity: Health Impact, Prevalence, Correlates and Interventions," *Psychology & Health* 32, no. 8 (2017): 942–75.

6. Steven H. Woolf and Paula Braveman, "The Social and Ecologic Determinants of Health," in *Contemporary Public Health: Principles, Practice and Policy,* ed. James W. Holsinger Jr. (Lexington: University Press of Kentucky, 2013), 25–46; Paula A. Braveman et al., "Health Disparities and Health Equity: The Issue Is Justice," *American Journal of Public*

Health 101, suppl. 1 (2011): S149–55; Olivia Egen et al., "Health and Social Conditions of the Poorest versus Wealthiest Counties in the United States," *American Journal of Public Health* 107, no. 1 (2017): 130–35.

7. Christopher J. L. Murray et al., "Eight Americas: Investigating Mortality Disparities across Races, Counties and Race–Counties in the United States," *PLoS Medicine* 3, no. 9 (2006): 1513–24.

8. Julie L. Marshall et al., *Creating a Culture of Health in Appalachia: Disparities and Bright Spots* (Washington, DC: Appalachian Regional Commission, 2017).

9. Steven H. Woolf, Derek A. Chapman, and F. Douglas Scutchfield, "Geographic Health Disparities in Kentucky: Starting a Conversation about Local Solutions," *Frontiers in Public Health Services and Systems Research* 5, no. 3 (2016): 1–8.

10. County Health Rankings, "What and Why We Rank," http://www.countyhealthrankings.org/explore-health-rankings/what-and-why-we-rank.

11. Michael Hendryx, Leah Wolfe, Juhua Luo, and Bo Webb, "Self-reported Cancer Rates in Two Rural Areas of West Virginia with and without Mountaintop Coal Mining," *Journal of Community Health* 37, no. 2 (2012): 320–27.

12. Anne Case and Angus Deaton, "Rising Morbidity and Mortality in Midlife among White Non-Hispanic Americans in the 21st Century," *Proceedings of the National Academy of Sciences of the United States of America* 112, no. 49 (2015): 15078–83; Michael Meit, Megan Heffernan, Erin Tanenbaum, and Topher Hoffmann, *Final Report: Appalachian Diseases of Despair* (Washington, DC: Appalachian Regional Commission, 2017).

2

Appalachia

An Introduction to the Region

RON R. ROACH

> Appalachia is a place, a people, an idea, a culture, and it exists as much in the mind and imagination as on the map. While it can be defined in any number of ways depending upon the person defining it, its story is rich in everything that makes human history exciting and compelling.
>
> Richard Straw, "Appalachian History"

For more than two centuries, scholars have struggled to define Appalachia. The first comprehensive study of the region was undertaken by John C. Campbell and Olive Dame Campbell, who came to the Appalachians as missionary educators early in the twentieth century. Unlike many outsiders who were drawn to work in the mountains, the Campbells were convinced that they should try to learn the true character of the place and its people. John obtained a grant to fund an extensive field survey that would provide real data about the region, based on an "impartial but sympathetic study" of "the mountaineer and his environment." In 1908–1909 the Campbells traveled by rail, wagon, and horseback through the mountains of North Carolina, Tennessee, and Kentucky, surveying communities as they went, and they discovered that the region was not as simple as they had been led to believe. In John's landmark study *The Southern Highlander and His Homeland* (1921), which Olive completed after his death, Campbell stated that he had first come to Appalachia confident "in that comprehensive knowledge which frequently characterizes a limited acquaintance with the subject." However, after experiencing the place firsthand and getting to know many of its residents, he famously concluded that Appalachia was "a land of promise, a land of romance, and a land about which, perhaps, more things are known that are not true than of any part of our country."[1]

Though written a century ago, Campbell's words still ring true today. Appalachia has long been a place of contradictions and the object of many competing definitions; it has periodically been "rediscovered" and subjected to endless misperceptions and stereotypes by the mass media of successive generations. Even today, the public is bombarded with a steady stream of "reality" television shows, drama series, novels, and horror films, all of which compete to position Appalachia and its residents as a dangerous "other," forever outside the American mainstream.

One of the latest examples of the rediscovery of Appalachia followed the 2016 presidential election, when journalists and pundits descended on the region and, in their attempt to explain why so many mountain residents had voted for Donald Trump, often resurrected the old stereotypes that have dehumanized and demeaned Appalachian residents. As historian Ron Eller observed, "Falling back on images of racism, religion, gun rights, ignorance, and anti-intellectualism, a few initial responses to Trump's victory reinforced the myth of Appalachia as a 'taker' region whose residents simply deserved what they would get from the new Trump administration." All this confirms what Jeff Biggers wrote in *The United States of Appalachia:* "Few regions in the United States confound and fascinate Americans like Appalachia. No other region has been so misrepresented by the mass media." Appalachia continues to fascinate and confound, and although many still believe they know things about the place, these things may not be true at all.[2]

Attempts to Map the Region

One of the reasons Appalachia has confounded observers is that it can be defined in very different ways depending on whether one approaches the region geographically, politically, economically, or culturally. The very name *Appalachia* is, to some degree, a reflection of this difficulty. Although indigenous peoples have inhabited the mountains for at least 12,000 years, the first Europeans to document their travel through the region were the members of Hernando de Soto's Spanish expedition, who journeyed through the mountains of present-day South Carolina, North Carolina, Tennessee, Georgia, and Alabama in 1540. Although we have no indication that de Soto or his men used the term, the name "Apalchen" appeared on a 1562 map by Spanish cartographer Diego Gutierrez. It is believed that the name was a distortion of the name of the Apalachee people, whom the Spanish had encountered and fought with in northern Florida. French mapmaker Jacques Le Moyne was the first to clearly apply the name to the mountain range itself ("Montes Apalatci"), on a 1564 map.[3]

The most clear-cut definition of the region is perhaps the geological one, as it relies on identifying the extent of the mountains themselves. Even here, however, there are differing opinions as to exactly where the mountains begin and end and which subranges to include. The most common approach defines the full extent of the Appalachian range as stretching from Alabama to

Newfoundland, a distance of nearly 2,500 miles. In addition to their impressive expanse, the Appalachians are among the most ancient mountains in the world—more than 480 million years old. They were formed through a series of massive tectonic plate collisions and ensuing erosions that saw the mountains soar to heights comparable to the modern Himalayas before receding to their present scale.

Today's Appalachian Mountains comprise a number of smaller ranges, such as the Blue Ridge, Allegheny, Cumberland, and Great Smoky Mountains, as well as an extensive system of parallel valleys, ridges, and plateaus. According to the US Geological Survey, the Appalachians span five geologic provinces in the United States: Appalachian Basin, Blue Ridge Mountains, Piedmont Province, Adirondack Province, and New England Province. Indeed, one of the most dominant features of the Appalachians is not a mountain at all but the Great Valley that leads from Pennsylvania, through Virginia, and deep into Tennessee.[4]

The mountains are also renowned for their powerful rivers, natural beauty, and biological diversity. According to biologist Charlotte Muir, the southern Appalachians are "one of the most biologically diverse regions in the temperate world . . . in terms of both the variety of different species and the abundance of each species." Some species of salamander and fungus have higher levels of diversity in the southern Appalachians than anywhere else, and the region boasts more than 100 native trees, 1,400 flowering plants, and 500 moss and fern species. Nearly 10,000 total species have been confirmed, and more are still being discovered.[5]

One of the first naturalists to record observations of the region was William Bartram, during his famous expedition through the southeastern colonies in 1773–1777. In 1775, during the early days of the American Revolution, Bartram traveled to Cherokee country in what is now upstate South Carolina and southwestern North Carolina. Like so many before and since, he was awestruck by the natural beauty he found there. As he arrived at the major Cherokee town of Cowee, north of present-day Franklin, North Carolina, Bartram wrote the following words, which resonate today:

> I arrived at Cowe [sic] about noon; this settlement is esteemed the capital town; it is situated on the bases of the hills on both sides of the river, near to its bank, and here terminates the great vale of Cowe, exhibiting one of the most charming natural mountainous landscapes perhaps any where to be seen; ridges of hills rising grand and sublimely one above and beyond another, some boldly and majestically advancing into the verdant plain, their feet bathed with the silver flood of the Tanase, whilst

others far distant, veiled in blue mists, sublimely mount aloft, with yet greater majesty lift up their pompous crests and overlook vast regions.[6]

Given the expanse of the Appalachian Mountains, it is not surprising that there have been so many attempts to define the boundaries of the region. One of the earliest was that by Berea College president William Goodell Frost, who in 1895 defined the region as 194 counties in nine states from West Virginia south to Alabama. The Campbells offered a similar map in 1921, with the flanks of the area expanded to include 254 counties, and called the region the "Southern Highlands."[7]

The most consequential attempt to define the region, however, came with the establishment of the Appalachian Regional Commission (ARC) in 1965. Formed as part of President Lyndon Johnson's War on Poverty, the ARC initially designated 360 counties in eleven states as part of the Appalachian region; this was later expanded to include counties in New York and Mississippi. Whereas Frost and the Campbells were interested primarily in cultural factors, the ARC map is a political designation, based largely on economic considerations and on collaboration between the federal and state governments. Consequently, some counties that were not traditionally considered part of Appalachia were included, while others were omitted. The list of ARC-designated counties has expanded gradually over the years so that it now contains 420 counties in thirteen states (figure 2.1).[8]

Today, although most students of the region acknowledge the benefits of the ARC designation and the resources and collaboration it encourages, they also recognize that, historically and culturally, the traditional core of Appalachia is composed of the Central and Southern subregions. Richard Straw, for example, writes, "for most who work in the region, [Appalachia] is the area of the United States that is situated mostly in the Southern mountains . . . generally made up of a core area: West Virginia, southwestern Virginia, eastern Kentucky, eastern Tennessee, western North Carolina, and the northern mountains of Georgia." At the same time, scholars emphasize the great complexity and local differences that exist across the region and admit that regional boundaries are imprecise. As John Alexander Williams notes, Appalachia is "a zone where diverse groups have interacted with one another and with a set of regional and subregional environments over time." Williams acknowledges the ARC designation of the larger region but, like Straw, identifies a traditional core area. Comparing the six most influential twentieth-century definitions of Appalachia, Williams delineates what he calls Core Appalachia, Consensus Appalachia, and Loose Appalachia. Consensus Appalachia, for example, contains 211 counties from Alabama to West Virginia (figure 2.2). Thus, despite

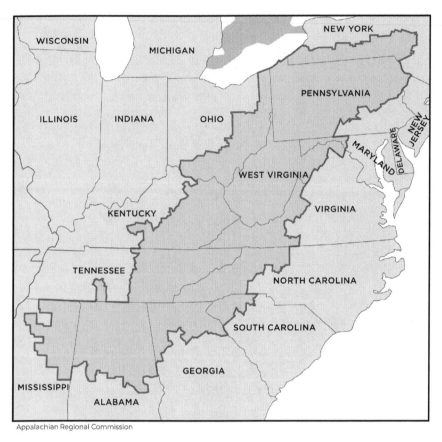

Appalachian Regional Commission

Figure 2.1. Appalachian region served by the ARC. (*Source:* ARC, 2021)

the existence of a rough consensus concerning the historical core of Appalachia, the exact boundaries remain elusive and ever shifting.⁹

However its physical boundaries are defined, all agree that the region is vast: the ARC-defined region stretches more than 1,000 miles north to south and encompasses more than 200,000 square miles. Its population exceeds 25 million; if it were a state, it would be the third largest in the nation. The region contains outstanding natural resources and wilderness areas, including more than 5 million acres of national forest; it has many rural communities but also encompasses numerous larger cities and metropolitan areas, including Birmingham, Knoxville and the Tri-Cities (Johnson City–Kingsport–Bristol), Charleston (West Virginia), and Pittsburgh.

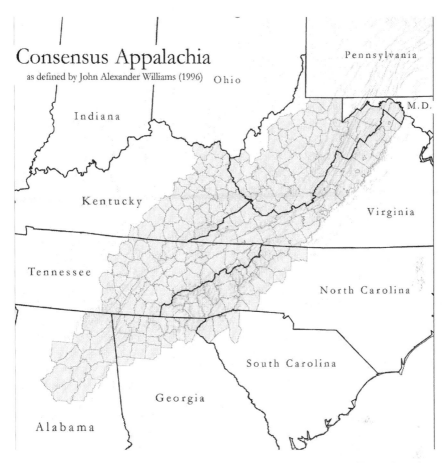

Figure 2.2. Consensus Appalachia according to John Alexander Williams (1996).
(*Source:* Stewart Scales, Emily Satterwhite, and Abigail August, "Mapping
Appalachia's Boundaries: Historiographic Overview and Digital Collection,"
Journal of Appalachian Studies 24, no. 1 [Spring 2018]: 89–100; Stewart Scales,
Emily Satterwhite, and Abigail August, Mapping Appalachia: A Digital Collection,
May 2018, https://www.mapappalachia.geography.vt.edu/. Used with permission.)

Another obvious fact is that the Appalachian Mountains are the most
dominant geographic feature east of the Rockies, as revealed by a glance at a
topographical map of the United States. Though relatively modest in height
compared with many mountain ranges, the Appalachians formed a formidable
barrier before the advent of modern transportation. It is easy to understand
why the mountains have exerted such an influence over ecology, settlement,
migration, culture, economics, and warfare through the centuries. One can also

appreciate why Washington Irving and Edgar Allan Poe suggested in the mid-1800s (though probably satirically) that the United States of America should be renamed the United States of Alleghenia or the United States of Appalachia. They reasoned that this would honor the central and unifying geographic feature of the new nation, while allowing it to keep using the initials USA.[10]

Historical Overview

The Appalachian Mountains have seen many successive waves of human exploration, settlement, and migration. The long valleys, rivers, and gaps through the mountains have always been natural thoroughfares for both animals and people, and many of the earliest human paths simply followed existing buffalo traces. Indeed, the buffalo, or American bison, was common in the region and very much in evidence when the first Europeans settled there. Archaeological evidence indicates that humans were first present in the region as hunter-gatherers at least 12,000 years ago and that by about 1300 BC there was a diverse population of indigenous peoples. From about AD 800 to 1600, the remarkable Mississippian and associated cultures, such as the Fort Ancient, flourished in the mountains. Evidence of their impressive civilization can be seen in the massive earthen mounds and exquisite artifacts they left behind, such as the Etowah Mound site in northern Georgia. Extensive trade routes existed throughout the region at this time, connecting the towns of Appalachia with inhabitants as far away as the Gulf coast and the Great Lakes.

When the de Soto expedition passed through the southern Appalachians in 1540, it encountered the remnants of the declining Mississippian culture and the beginnings of the Cherokee ascendancy. In 1567, nearly two decades before the first English colony at Roanoke Island, the Spanish attempted to establish a presence in the Appalachians, building a fort at Joara, near present-day Morganton, North Carolina. However, the Spanish were quite belligerent toward the indigenous inhabitants, and the garrison was nearly wiped out in less than two years. Another deadly legacy of the Spanish expeditions was the introduction of diseases for which the indigenous peoples had no immunity, leading to widespread death and a devastating decline in population, which likely hastened the end of the Mississippian culture.[11]

By the 1600s, the Cherokee, who spoke an Iroquoian language, were the dominant group in the southern Appalachians. Other indigenous peoples in the region included the Creek to the south, the Catawba to the east, and the Shawnee to the north. The Cherokee had a strong spiritual connection to the mountains; they considered their homeland to be the center of the world, gifted to them by the Great Spirit above. James Mooney, the earliest ethnographer to study the Cherokee, described them as the first "mountaineers of the South." They controlled nearly 40,000 acres of land from the Ohio River into northern Georgia. The Cherokee developed a rich culture centered around their villages, located along rivers in the mountains. They had a thriving agriculture, managed by the women, and engaged in hunting and gathering, managed by the men. At its height, the Cherokee nation numbered between 30,000 and 35,000 inhabitants concentrated in three subregions: the Lower Towns, in today's upstate South Carolina and northeastern Georgia; the Middle Towns, in southwestern North Carolina; and the Overhill Towns of southeastern Tennessee.[12]

In the late 1700s European settlers began to push into the region from the east, and war between the British and French empires spilled onto the frontier. This led to increasing conflict between the Europeans and the indigenous peoples, as Britain and France recruited various tribes as allies. By the 1760s, the British had defeated both the French and the Cherokee in the French and Indian War, although conflict between the Cherokee and the settlers continued for many years, especially during the American Revolution. Meanwhile, the tide of colonists crossing the mountains kept growing. The major migration route for the settlers was from Pennsylvania down the Great Valley into Virginia, then into North Carolina or present-day Tennessee.

The Cherokee, more than any of the other southeastern Indians, adopted the cultural practices of the European settlers. In 1821 Sequoya invented a syllabary for writing the Cherokee language; seven years later, the first Native American newspaper, the *Cherokee Phoenix,* was published in Cherokee and English. The Cherokee nation even adopted a constitutional government modeled after that of the United States, but nothing stemmed the relentless advance of white settlers. By the 1830s, the Cherokee lands had been reduced to a portion of northern Georgia (with a capital at New Echota), southwestern North Carolina, and eastern Tennessee. The ongoing thirst for land, the discovery of gold in northern Georgia, and the policies of President Andrew Jackson culminated in the forced removal of most Cherokee to modern-day Oklahoma in 1838–1839, with only a small remnant remaining in the Qualla Boundary in North Carolina; today, their descendants constitute the Eastern Band of the Cherokee Indians. Tragically, of the approximately 18,000 Cherokee forced to relocate, at least 4,000 perished on what came to be known as the Trail of Tears.[13]

Black Appalachians were an important minority group in the Appalachian region from the very beginning of European exploration. African slaves were part of both Spanish and French exploration parties, and at least one enslaved man escaped from the de Soto expedition to cohabitate with the Cherokee. As William H. Turner notes, "blacks were in the region long before the major migrations of white settlers took place," and "black Appalachians were some of America's *first* blacks—appearing almost a century before the landing at Jamestown." Due to the absence of large plantations in the mountains, slavery was not practiced on a vast scale, but it was present to varying degrees throughout the southern mountains, practiced by both white settlers and Cherokee. In addition, some free blacks settled in the region. Thus, in the years leading up to the Civil War, the number of blacks in the region gradually increased, and by 1860, they constituted about 10 percent of the population. After the war, an increasing number of blacks moved to the mountains to work in the coalfields, on the railroads, and in other industries. The largest migration of blacks into the region took place between 1900 and 1930, as many blacks relocated from the Deep South into coal-mining country.[14]

The white settlers who made their homes in the southern Appalachians were of various European origins, mostly Scots-Irish and English, with smaller numbers of Germans, Welsh, French, Dutch, and Swiss. Although the exact figures are unknown, as many as 40 percent of the earliest settlers in parts of the southern mountains were likely Scots-Irish from Ulster in Northern Ireland. At least 250,000 Scots-Irish immigrated to the American colonies during the 1700s, and large numbers migrated to the mountains from earlier settlements in Pennsylvania, Virginia, and North Carolina. Farther north in the region, the percentage of German settlers was higher, and by the late 1800s, sizable numbers of southern and eastern Europeans had immigrated to the coalfields and to the growing industrial cities of Central and Northern Appalachia.[15]

Although the Scots-Irish influence in Southern Appalachia was certainly significant, it has sometimes been overemphasized to the point that other groups have been overlooked. It is clear, however, that the early settlers in the region were hardy, independent, ambitious, and adventurous. The first colonists who crossed the Blue Ridge and settled in the Watauga area of northeastern Tennessee did so in defiance of King George's Proclamation of 1763 and risked conflict with the Cherokee and Shawnee. In 1772 these pioneers created the Watauga Association, believed by many to be the American colonists' first attempt to form an independent government, although the area was quickly confirmed as part of North Carolina. During the American Revolution, it was these pioneers who crossed back over the mountains to defeat Patrick Ferguson's loyalist army at the Battle of King's Mountain, which Thomas Jefferson described as the turning point in the Revolution.

After the Revolution, during the new nation's first decades, a vibrant frontier culture developed in Appalachia. As white Appalachians, black Appalachians, and Native Americans commingled, each group contributed to a common way of life. This frontier lifestyle was largely agrarian, based on hunting, farming, gathering, and herding; it was centered around largely self-sufficient homesteads and reliant on the vast commons of the forest landscape. A strong agricultural economy and early timber and mining industries developed, with active trade routes and the exportation of agricultural goods to the more populous settlements in the Piedmont and coastal areas. Some consider this to be the region's strongest economic period in comparison to the rest of the country.[16]

The Civil War brought an abrupt end to this strong mountain economy and left the region in a desperate situation. Politically, residents of the mountain counties were split: in some counties, a majority supported the Confederacy, while in others, particularly in the mountains of Virginia and eastern Tennessee, a majority supported the Union. With the exception of the campaigns around Chattanooga and in northern Georgia, few large-scale battles took place in the mountains. However, the region was shattered by Union raiders and Confederate home guards, internecine strife and brutal reprisals, severe deprivation on the home front, and the destruction of railroads and bridges. Moreover, thousands of young men were killed or wounded, and the economy was left in ruins. After the war, developers, investors, and magnates began to discover and exploit the rich resources of the region. The rapid industrialization of the country created a growing demand for coal and timber, and entrepreneurs swept into the mountains, where these resources were in ready supply. These industries spurred the rapid expansion of railroads into the region, resulting in swift communication with the rest of the country. Thus began a cycle of large-scale absentee ownership and extractive industry that marginalized and displaced many of the region's inhabitants, altered economic and social structures, and left indelible marks on Appalachia to this day. As Steven Stoll notes in *Ramp Hollow: The Ordeal of Appalachia*, the "scramble for Appalachia" had begun, with efforts to "clear-cut the forests and dig out the coal" as the region experienced merely a "shadow" of the Industrial Revolution taking place elsewhere in the country. By 1930, as much as 80 percent of the land in southern West Virginia was owned by coal, oil, and railroad companies, virtually ending the traditional practice of common grazing lands. The Appalachian family farm had been devastated: in 1880 the average farm contained 187 acres of land; by 1930, it was only 76 acres.[17]

Cataclysmic world events in the early twentieth century—World War I, the Great Depression, and World War II—exerted a great influence on the economy, way of life, and, consequently, population growth and decline in Appalachia. As Paul Salstrom writes, "As of 1840, southern Appalachia figured as one of the most self-sufficient regions of the United States. By 1940 it had become one of the *least* self-sufficient regions." Large numbers of people moved out of Appalachia, whether in search of jobs or to serve in the war effort. These migrations and those that followed World War II—sometimes called the "Southern

Diaspora"—significantly affected the American South and the southern Appalachian Mountains. Between 1900 and 1980, around 20 million southerners, both black and white, left the South to settle in western, midwestern, and northern cities. Many Appalachians moved to towns and cities on the periphery of the region, particularly in Ohio and in the textile towns of the southern Piedmont. Sizable communities of Appalachians were also established in many cities well outside the region, such as Chicago and Detroit. These emigrants not only encountered prejudice and discrimination because of their Appalachian roots but, along with other southerners, also had a profound impact on the development of American religion, music, politics, and popular culture in the late twentieth century. The cycle of out-migration, in-migration, and shuttle migration continues in Appalachia with varying intensity to the present day.[18]

Alongside these events, the nation's hunger for coal to fuel the economy and its war efforts, as well as the growing demand for household electric power, propelled coal mining to replace logging as the largest extractive industry in the region, particularly in Central Appalachia. A major driver of this economic expansion was the Tennessee Valley Authority (TVA), which was founded in 1933 and had constructed sixteen hydroelectric dams by 1944. The TVA brought thousands of jobs to the region, extended electricity to rural households across the South, helped prevent flooding and soil erosion, and lured other industries to the cities of Southern Appalachia. However, the TVA also displaced thousands of residents from their homes, and its dams, man-made lakes, and power plants and the resulting pollution changed the Appalachian landscape. Entire towns, hundreds of farms, and many irreplaceable Native American historical sites were submerged forever.

The early decades of the twentieth century also saw the formation of governmental organizations and recreational areas that would have a profound impact on the Appalachian region. In 1905 the US Forest Service was founded, with Gifford Pinchot as its first director. Pinchot had earlier served as chief forester for George Vanderbilt's Biltmore forests near Asheville, North Carolina. By the 1920s, the Forest Service had established four national forests in the southern mountains and acquired more than 2 million acres of forestland in the Appalachians, 70 percent of which had been severely affected by burning or clear-cutting. In 1921 Benton MacKaye proposed an Appalachian Trail to run through the mountains from Georgia to Maine. The full trail, which was completed in 1937, is now 2,192 miles long and is used by more than 3 million people each year. In 1916 the National Park Service was formed; by the 1930s, it had begun construction on major parks and scenic drives in Appalachia, including Great Smoky Mountains National Park (1934) and the Blue Ridge Parkway (1935). These federal projects inevitably had an impact on the environment and, like the TVA projects, displaced many residents. Yet overall, they played a vital role in conserving Appalachian wilderness areas.[19]

Events during the 1960s had a profound impact on both the popular conception of Appalachia and its future development. Early in the decade, the public consciousness of the need to mitigate poverty in America was enhanced. In 1962, for example, Michael Harrington published *The Other America: Poverty in the United States,* in which he argued that American society perpetuated a culture of poverty among its poorest members. This book influenced John F. Kennedy, whose hard-fought Democratic primary campaign in West Virginia in 1960 had shone a spotlight on the region's economic plight. Alongside the antipoverty movement was the growing conservation movement, energized by such works as Rachel Carson's *Silent Spring* (1962). In 1963 Kentucky attorney and activist Harry Caudill brought both these movements to bear on Appalachia in *Night Comes to the Cumberlands,* a surprise best seller that resonated with messages about both poverty and the environment. He vehemently condemned the practices of the coal industry and called for the formation of a federal organization to assist the region, modeled on the TVA. Although Caudill's book has been criticized for inadequate research and the use of cultural stereotypes, it had a profound impact on public perceptions of the region. More than any other work, it cemented in the national consciousness the image of Appalachia as a region of desperate poverty that demanded outside intervention. It also helped precipitate a flood of television and photographic images, journalistic reports, and other writings focused on coal mining and the poorest parts of the mountains. In 1964 President Lyndon Johnson proclaimed the national War on Poverty, which led to the creation of the ARC in 1965.[20]

The 1960s also introduced Appalachian studies as a field of inquiry in colleges and universities. The concept of regional studies, in which multidisciplinary approaches are used to study and promote development in a particular region, grew out of the regional science movement founded in the 1950s by economist Walter Isard. In the late 1960s Helen M. Lewis started the first overtly Appalachian studies courses at Clinch Valley College in Virginia. Within a few years, numerous institutions were offering classes focused on the region, and several had founded academic centers for research and service. What is now called the Appalachian Studies Association (ASA) was founded in 1978, and although it is led primarily by academics, it has a wide range of constituents from the region, including artists, activists, and other citizens. From the 1970s to the present, the ARC and ASA have been two of the leaders in efforts to provide accurate data about Appalachia and to propose solutions to its challenges.

The last decades of the twentieth century saw great changes in Appalachia. The ARC spurred investment in infrastructure across the region, encouraging better highways, higher incomes, decreased poverty rates, greater economic diversification, and improved education levels. However, population and economic growth varied. The population in Appalachia grew at a slower rate than in the rest of the country, and most of that growth was in the southern part of the region. Central and Northern Appalachia experienced much slower population growth, and some counties even saw a decrease due to the continued decline of coal mining and manufacturing. Coal mining in the region reached its peak in 1940, when more than 130,000 workers were employed in West Virginia alone. However, these numbers decreased dramatically due to mechanization and the rise of surface mining. In the 1990s the deregulation of global trade policies, particularly by the North American Free Trade Agreement (NAFTA), was a major factor in the widespread closure of manufacturing plants across the region and in numerous cities on the periphery of the region, which had been traditional destinations for Appalachian out-migrants seeking employment.[21]

Prevailing Misconceptions

The 1960s narrative of poverty-stricken Appalachia was accompanied by a renewed display of old stereotypes in popular culture, encouraged by television series such as *The Beverly Hillbillies* and the infamous portrayal of mountain residents in the film *Deliverance* (1973). In the decades that followed, several common misconceptions, many of which had been present in earlier generations, were routinely promulgated and are still widely evident today.

Isolation and Backwardness

Appalachians have long been depicted as completely isolated, trapped in the past, and bypassed by the modern world. This belief appears as early as the accounts of Virginia planter and surveyor William Byrd II in the 1720s, and it was firmly ensconced by the writers of the local color, or literary regionalism, movement of the late 1800s. In 1899 William Goodell Frost promoted this stereotype in the *Atlantic* magazine, describing Appalachian residents as "our contemporary ancestors":

> At the close of the Revolutionary War there were about two and one half million people in the American colonies. Today there are in the Southern mountains approximately the same number of people—Americans for four and five generations—who are living to all intents and purposes in the conditions of the colonial times! . . . Their remoteness is by no means measured by the mere distance in miles. It is a longer journey from northern Ohio to eastern Kentucky than from America to Europe; for one day's ride brings us into the eighteenth century.[22]

This view, one of the most pervasive and denigrating myths about Appalachians, has been widely repeated in both academic writing and popular culture.

In the mid-twentieth century British historian Arnold Toynbee wrote, "In fact, the Appalachian 'mountain people' to-day are no better than barbarians. They have relapsed into illiteracy and witchcraft. They suffer from poverty, squalor and ill-health. . . . [They] represent the melancholy spectacle of a people who have acquired civilization and then lost it." This stereotype was also a central theme of the rediscovery of Appalachia in the 1960s, figuring prominently in Kentucky minister Jack Weller's widely read *Yesterday's People: Life in Contemporary Appalachia* (1965) and in Bruce and Nancy Roberts's *Where Time Stood Still: A Portrait of Appalachia*. The latter wrote: "For many years the lack of roads and the natural difficulties of travel through mountain areas resulted in isolation for those who lived there. Generation after generation of children grew up, married, and raised their own families, never leaving the immediate area of their birth. Listening to the voices of the mountain people, one still hears traces of an Elizabethan accent like faint echoes from their pioneer past."[23]

Contrary to this stereotype, Appalachians were never completely isolated, even though the mountainous terrain made travel to rural areas difficult in the past. Further, it does not follow that these people were any more backward, morally depraved, or unintelligent (as was asserted) than those living in other parts of the country. In addition, the region's great geographic diversity ensured that many areas of Appalachia were not only well connected to other regions but also major trade and migration routes. This was not surprising: before the earliest European exploration, the mountains were traversed by an extensive network of Native American trails, including well-traveled interregional corridors such as the Great Indian Warpath, the Catawba Trail, and the Trading Path. Most of these paths later developed into wagon roads and turnpikes, which became the basis for many of today's major highways. It has been well documented that even in colonial times, the region was economically connected to the rest of the nation. Ronald L. Lewis wrote, "As early as 1800 cattle and hogs were being driven from the Carolina mountains to markets in Charleston, Savannah, Norfolk, and Philadelphia." By the late 1800s, railroads crisscrossed the region, providing easy access to northern, midwestern, and eastern cities. By the 1920s, the rising popularity of automobiles ensured that paved roads were being built in many mountain areas. Since 1965, one of the ARC's priorities has been to spur the construction of transportation infrastructure in the mountains, and today, modern highways crisscross the region.[24]

In 2006, countering the "backwardness" stereotype, historian and journalist Jeff Biggers wrote *The United States of Appalachia*, documenting many examples of Appalachian men and women who were at the vanguard of important events and advances in American history such as the Revolution; the abolitionist movement; the development of American musical forms, including blues and country; the creation of modern journalism; and the civil rights movement. Biggers concluded: "This is Appalachia's best-kept secret. Far from being a 'strange land with a peculiar people,' the mountains and hills have been a stage for some of the most quintessential and daring American experiences of innovation, rebellion, and social change."[25]

The Elizabethan dialect myth noted earlier is often cited as proof of the isolation stereotype. However, this claim has been thoroughly discredited by linguistic scholars on several counts: the Elizabethan period ended more than 150 years before the first large-scale British settlement of the Appalachian region, most of the earliest settlers in the mountains had already been living in the American colonies for at least a generation, and a linguistic analysis of contemporary Appalachian speech did not find the reputed preservation of Elizabethan language. Despite these findings, this myth still resurfaces today, as recently as a 2017 article in *Appalachian Magazine*.[26]

Racial Homogeneity

Another widely held misconception is that Appalachia is populated entirely by white people of British descent. In 1901 Ellen Churchill Semple wrote, "In these isolated communities . . . we find the purest Anglo-Saxon stock in all the United States." As late as 2005, the Library of Congress's standard catalog heading for Appalachian people was "Mountain Whites"; Appalachian State University professor Fred Hay led the fight to get it changed. While it is true that Appalachia as a whole has a higher percentage of whites than the national average and that many rural areas in the region have very small minority populations, minority groups have always had a significant but often over-looked presence. By the colonial period, whites, blacks, and Native Americans were living side by side in the mountains, developing a way of life comprising elements from each culture. Patterns of construction, agriculture, hunting, foodways, medicine, religious beliefs, and music exhibited contributions from the disparate groups inhabiting the region. Since the mid-1800s, blacks have been the largest minority group in Appalachia and have had an immense impact on its history and culture. By 1900, the total population of the Appalachian region had grown to 4.76 million people, 14 percent of whom were black. In addition to blacks, many immigrants from Ireland, Wales, and eastern and southern Europe flocked to the coalfields in the late nineteenth and early twentieth centuries, and some estimate that immigrants accounted for

50 percent or more of the mining workforce in Northern Appalachia during this period. Minorities continue to play a major role in Appalachia today; in 2017, of the total population of 25.6 million, racial and ethnic minorities made up 18.1 percent (9.2 percent black, 5.1 percent Hispanic and Latino, 3.8 percent other).[27]

Culture of Poverty

After being popularized by Harrington in the early 1960s, the culture of poverty theory was quickly taken up by others, including anthropologist Oscar Lewis and writers such as Caudill and Weller, who applied the concept to Appalachia. However, this theory has now been largely discredited. One criticism is that the theory embraces negative stereotyping and tends to blame the poor for their problems, positing that if they just changed their culture, they could escape poverty. The theory also assumes that culture is static from generation to generation, and rigid cultural traits are replicated. More recent theorists recognize that culture is not static, that behaviors do not always accurately reflect cultural values and attitudes, and that other structural and societal factors can exert great influence on individuals.[28]

Criticism of the theory has not prevented the continued perception that a widespread culture of poverty is to blame for conditions in Appalachia. In 2016 J. D. Vance's *Hillbilly Elegy: A Memoir of a Family and Culture in Crisis* became a runaway best seller and was embraced by observers from both ends of the political spectrum, who latched on to it as a Rosetta stone for deciphering Appalachia. Not since Caudill's *Night Comes to the Cumberlands* had a book about Appalachia garnered so much attention in the national media. Vance's book raises valid points about drug abuse and about the challenges faced by first-generation college students, and he inspired many with his personal success story, but the book has major flaws. For one thing, Vance is not a native of the Appalachian region, although his grandparents were. In addition, he presents the book as a memoir but makes sweeping generalizations about the region based on limited anecdotal evidence. Commentators looking for a fast explanation or perhaps validation of their own preconceived notions accepted these generalizations with little question. Vance also resurrects the culture of poverty model, seeming to blame the Appalachian people for their problems. Appalachian residents, scholars, and activists vigorously refuted *Hillbilly Elegy* and protested its knee-jerk acceptance as a definitive work on the region, a response that ignored decades of research and the deeper issues underlying the region's problems and its residents' political disaffection. Despite this, Vance's book continues to be accepted by many.[29]

Culture of Violence

In recent years, several popular books have claimed to identify regional cultures in North America that supposedly persisted from the original European settlers, such as David Hackett Fisher's *Albion's Seed: Four British Folkways in America,* Colin Woodard's *American Nations: A History of the Eleven Rival Regional Cultures of North America,* and Jim Webb's *Born Fighting: How the Scots-Irish Shaped America.* A common theme in these works is the assertion that the Appalachian people have preserved a culture of feuding and violence brought from the British Isles by herders from the Scottish Highlands, Ulster (Northern Ireland), and the English border region. This thesis was also popularized by psychologists Richard Nisbett and Dov Cohen in *Culture of Honor: The Psychology of Violence in the South.* However, the culture of violence stereotype has been exaggerated and unfairly paints the entire region as a savage and dangerous place. The existence of violence in the region is not surprising, since Appalachia was the first frontier of the nascent United States and, consequently, was on the front line of conflicts among settlers, British and French forces, and Native Americans well into the nineteenth century. However, the feuding stereotype holds that there is an inherent predisposition toward violence because of older cultural traits that have been passed on. This belief clearly relies on the same problematic assumptions of a static culture and centuries of isolation noted earlier. In addition, publications advancing the culture of violence theory are based largely on generalizations and anecdotes, and Nisbett and Cohen's text has been strongly criticized for its faulty use of statistics and disregard of contradictory evidence.[30]

Altina Waller argues convincingly in *Feud: Hatfields, McCoys, and Social Change in Appalachia* that the feuds of Southern Appalachia were exaggerated by northern newspapers and local color writers during the late nineteenth century, often relying on the negative stereotype of a violent, backward culture. The most famous of the feuds, between the Hatfields and the McCoys, was transformed into a trope of popular media and has inspired an unending stream of representations in popular culture, including novels such as *The Trail of the Lonesome Pine;* comic strips such as *Lil' Abner* and *Snuffy Smith;* countless films and television shows such as *The Andy Griffith Show* and the (historically inaccurate) Kevin Costner miniseries *Hatfields and McCoys,* broadcast on the History Channel in 2012; and tourist attractions such as the Hatfield and McCoy Dinner Feud in Pigeon Forge, Tennessee, and the Hatfield–McCoy trails in West Virginia. Although terrible violence was committed during the Hatfield–McCoy feud, Waller has demonstrated that nearly every facet of the myth was inflated: the two families were not definitively divided (there were

McCoys on the Hatfield side, and vice versa), numerous participants were not members of either family, the violence lasted only twelve years and only twelve people were killed, and much of the conflict stemmed from economic rivalries rather than an inherent thirst for violence. Nevertheless, the feud stereotype is now the stuff of legend, and the tourism bureaus of both Kentucky and West Virginia use it to boost revenue.[31]

Romanticization of Appalachia

In contrast to the many negative images of the region, some have promoted an idealistic vision of Appalachia as a sanctuary from the modern world, filled with yeoman farmers living a pastoral life. Biggers called this misconception "Pristine Appalachia," which imagines a place of "unspoiled mountains and hills along the Appalachian Trail." Unfortunately, as Biggers points out, this rosy view overlooks the "centuries of warfare, the wholesale destruction of the virgin forests by the timber industry, and the continual bane of strip mining." Once again, the region's complexity is revealed, even in the contradictory stereotypes applied to it. The truth, of course, is somewhere in between.[32]

Stereotyping and Health Care

Most of the misperceptions discussed above have been adopted as stereotypes of Appalachian residents. Stereotypes, defined by psychologists as "qualities perceived to be associated with particular groups or categories of people," are a universal feature of human reasoning; everyone engages in stereotyping to some degree. Stereotyping becomes a problem, however, when it leads to prejudice and discrimination. Although much has been written about the validity of the common myths about Appalachia, until recently, little research has attempted to ascertain the actual effects of stereotypes on Appalachians. Similarly, only in the past twenty-five years have researchers begun to focus on how stereotypes influence health care. In the mid-1990s psychologists Claude Steele and Joshua Aronson were the first to identify the phenomenon of "stereotype threat"—a "disruptive psychological state that people experience when they feel at risk for confirming a negative stereotype associated with their social identity"—and to show its detrimental effects on health care. As Aronson and colleagues argued in 2013, "research confirms that health care providers stereotype their patients and that patients sense this bias and, as a result, feel dissatisfied with the care they receive. . . . The experience of stereotype threat has been shown to have direct negative effects on physiological, psychological, and self-regulatory processes that can contribute to ill health." In addition, stereotype threat can lead to avoidance of care, impaired communication, and failure to adhere to treatment. Although further research is needed to determine the range of effects that stereotyping can have on the Appalachian population, health care providers can benefit from an increased awareness of stereotyping and should adopt strategies to minimize its potential harmful effects.[33]

Culture, Place, and Cultural Competency

The persistent misconceptions and stereotypes about Appalachia have complicated the study of local culture. It is commonly understood that there are cultural differences between regions and that, to varying degrees, localities have distinctive cultures. The question is: to what extent can one identify a distinctive culture for the Appalachian region? Not surprisingly, scholars have vigorously debated this issue.

There is a long tradition in the social sciences of studying regional and local cultures; however, such an analysis is difficult when dealing with a large, diverse region with inexact boundaries and extensive overlap with other regions. Also complicating the issue is the fact that approaches to the study of culture have shifted over time. In the first half of the twentieth century, most scholars viewed culture as the accumulated beliefs, values, and lifestyle of a particular group. We now recognize that the concept of culture is not quite so simple and that it involves interrelated systems, symbols, power structures, and symbolic actions that shift over time.[34]

In the quest to identify an Appalachian regional culture, views have generally veered between two extremes. On the one hand, the region has often been reduced to a list of static traits, an approach that overlooks the great diversity that exists across the region. On the other hand, some have argued that Appalachia is not a unique region at all; rather, it is an idea constructed by academics, writers, politicians, and other opinion makers from outside the region. Neither of these views provides a complete picture of the complexity of regional culture. A more useful approach is to simultaneously take account of the region's great diversity and the significant role played by ideas and symbols in the construction of regional concepts and identity, while at the same time recognizing the importance of a sense of place and local cultural differences.

Such a balanced, interdisciplinary process of inquiry would share many features with the "critical regionalism" methodology advocated by Douglas Reichert Powell and others, which focuses on the region "as a rich, complicated, and dynamic cultural construct rather than a static, stable geophysical entity." This approach considers how humans impart meaning to particular places through a number of processes; it also considers how a place is interconnected with broader regional, national, and global issues. Critical regionalism, in Powell's view, can lead beyond simplistic depictions of a region and provide the broader perspectives necessary to implement meaningful policies and actions that address endemic regional problems.[35]

Sense of Place

Numerous scholars have noted that a sense of place is an essential part of any study of Appalachian regional culture. A person's connection to a place and its cultural landscape plays a major role in the development of culture and identity. This emphasis has been shared by researchers in numerous disciplines. For example, philosopher Edward S. Casey pointed out that the word *culture* "goes back to Latin *colere*, 'to inhabit, care for, till, worship.' To be cultural, to have a culture, is to inhabit a place sufficiently intensely to cultivate it—to be responsible for it, to respond to it, to attend to it caringly. Where else but in particular places can culture take root?" Casey argued that a region is itself defined by places: particular places that have major traits in common despite the many differences within the region.[36]

Scholars now recognize that place matters and that our environment is linked to our physical, mental, and spiritual health. As physician Esther M. Sternberg demonstrates in *Healing Places: The Science of Place and Well-Being*, we have known for thousands of years that nature and place are important to healing; this knowledge now has a scientific basis as well. She writes, "Implicit in an understanding of the mind-body connection is an assumption that physical spaces that set the mind at ease can contribute to well-being, and those that trouble the emotions might foster illness."[37]

Dramatic natural landscapes such as mountains have always elicited a particularly strong sense of place in humans, as demonstrated by these places' important roles in religious traditions worldwide. Eighteenth-century philosophers such as Edmund Burke wrote of "the sublime," the overwhelming sense of awe and majesty we feel when confronted with a dramatic landscape. Robert MacFarlane, in *Mountains of the Mind*, observes, "When we look at a landscape, we do not see what is there, but largely what we think is there. We attribute qualities to a landscape which it does not intrinsically possess. . . . A disjunction between the imagined and the real is a characteristic of all human activities, but it finds one of its sharpest expressions in the mountains." Such responses are part of the complex process by which humans respond to the natural landscape and create a cultural landscape and sense of place.[38]

Local Culture

Following the methodology of critical regionalism and the concepts of place and placemaking, it follows that it is more useful to (1) think of regional cultures (plural) rather than one overarching regional culture; (2) consider the processes by which ideas of culture, place, and identity are created and inter-relate; and (3) focus on the level of local culture found in the subregions and communities within Greater Appalachia. As noted earlier, numerous scholars have described a traditional core of the Appalachian region, spanning from the West Virginia–Pennsylvania border south to northern Georgia and Alabama. Researchers focusing on this core area have repeatedly identi-fied broad demographic and cultural attributes that are typical of many inhab-itants. Susan Keefe, in *Appalachian Cultural Competency: A Guide for Medical, Mental Health, and Social Service Professionals,* followed this approach, citing her own research and more than twenty ethnographic studies to identify traditional cultural traits such as a distinctive linguistic dialect, a social struc-ture strongly based on kinship, local community as a source of identity and social organization, an independent Protestant religious heritage, and a strong sense of place. Similarly, many observers have described common characteris-tics of the traditional folklife and material culture of the core Appalachian region. Keefe correctly stressed, however, that "the existence of an Appala-chian cultural core does not imply the nonexistence of other, subdominant cultures in the region." Diverse ethnic and racial minority groups are also an important part of the region's population, and although these groups main-tain their own heritage, they also reflect and contribute to the traditional core culture.[39]

When attempting to define a broader regional culture, Keefe encountered the same difficulties as other researchers: although one can identify general cul-tural features of the traditional core of Appalachia, it is difficult to do this for the region as a whole. For one thing, the inhabitants share many cultural character-istics with the national culture and with the rural South, so cultural differences tend to be a matter of degree rather than kind. Finally, cultural traits—dialect being a prime example—can vary widely from place to place even within the core region.[40]

Intercultural Competence

Given these difficulties, how should health care providers respond to the com-plicated issue of Appalachian culture? Building on the approach of critical regionalism, on the importance of a sense of place and local culture, and on the growing literature about the role of stereotyping in health care, it is clear that providers can benefit from applying the principles of intercultural competence. Intercultural competence (known as cultural competence in some disciplines) is an ongoing process of developing awareness, attitudes, and communication skills to interact more effectively with people from other cultures or subcultures. As Keefe notes, "In the case of Appalachia, as in all others, there is no aspect of life that exists without cultural meaning. Appalachian people have their own way of looking at the world and acting in it. Those who hope to work successfully with them must learn to understand and appreciate these cultural differences."[41]

The importance of intercultural competence in health care was given a strong endorsement in 2000 when the US Department of Health and Human Services produced the first national standards for culturally and linguistically appropriate services (CLAS) in health and health care. There are now fifteen CLAS standards, the first of which is to "provide effective, equitable, under-standable, and respectful quality care and services that are responsive to diverse cultural health beliefs and practices, preferred languages, health literacy, and other communication needs." Although the CLAS standards largely focus on cultural differences based on race and ethnicity, they apply to all cultural differences and can be effectively utilized with cultures and subcultures within a region such as Appalachia. Moreover, intercultural competence has been recognized as "one of the most modifiable" factors contributing to inequities in health care, a fact that supports improved training in this area for health care providers and other professionals serving the region.[42]

Appalachia Today

The year 2015 marked the fiftieth anniversary of the ARC, a milestone that prompted several retrospective studies of the progress made over the past five decades. From its founding through 2013, the ARC and other federal, state, and local agencies invested more than $25 billion in the Appalachian region, and ARC investments attracted another $16 billion in leveraged private investments. On many socioeconomic measures, the Appalachian region made significant progress compared with the nation as a whole. However, such progress was not evenly distributed across the region, and significant challenges remain in many areas, as summarized in the following sections.[43]

Population

The overall population growth of Appalachia continues to lag behind that of the rest of the nation. From 2010 to 2017, for example, the US population increased by more than 5 percent, while that of Appalachia increased by only 1.4 percent. In fact, most of the region has lost population since 2010. Eight Appalachian states saw a decline in population during that period, and the decline was especially severe in Northern Appalachia. Population growth continues to be concentrated mainly in Southern Appalachia, with most of the growth occurring in counties near metropolitan areas, those that are attractive retirement destinations, and those near major universities.[44]

In terms of population, Appalachia remains more rural than the rest of the nation: 42 percent of Appalachians live in rural areas, compared with 20 percent nationally. However, the reverse of this statistic is usually overlooked: the majority of Appalachians live in urban areas, although they are much more likely to live in smaller urban centers than are urban residents elsewhere in the country. The region continues to experience the out-migration of adults between the ages of eighteen and thirty-five, contributing to the fact that most Appalachian counties have older populations than the national average. The region also continues to have a smaller percentage of minorities than the rest of the nation (18.6 versus 39.3 percent), although this number is increasing (up from 16.4 percent in 2010). Blacks continue to be the largest minority group (9.7 percent), but Hispanics and Latinos are still the fastest-growing minority group, accounting for 5.1 percent of the population (compared with 4.2 percent in 2010).[45]

Economic Measures

Appalachia's poverty rate has nearly been cut in half—from about 31 percent in 1960 to 16.3 percent in 2017. However, this is still higher than the national average of 14.6 percent. Income levels have increased in the region but are still substantially lower than in the country as a whole: in 2017 the median household income was $47,836 in Appalachia, or just 83 percent of the national average of $57,652. Pockets of severe economic struggle are still evident. In 2019 eighty-one counties, about one-fifth of the region, were categorized as economically distressed, and thirty-eight of those counties were in Kentucky.[46]

Unemployment rates have improved a great deal but are still slightly higher than the national average. In 1960 the Appalachian region's unemployment rate stood at 7.1 percent, more than 2 percentage points higher than the national rate of 5 percent. In 2017 the unemployment rate in Appalachia was 4.8 percent, compared with 4.4 percent in the nation. However, unemployment in some parts of the region, especially the coal-mining areas, is much worse. Overall, the unemployment rate stood at 7.3 percent in Central Appalachia, but it was even higher in some counties.[47]

Employment in manufacturing and mining has continued to decline in the region. Manufacturing jobs in Appalachia reached a peak of 2.2 million in 1979 but had fallen to only 1.2 million jobs by 2012. The sharp decrease in coal mining since 2000 has been driven by lower prices for natural gas, more rigorous environmental regulations, the closing of many coal-fired power plants, and a drop in international demand for US coal. In 2011 coal provided the fuel for more than 50 percent of electricity production in the United States, with natural gas accounting for about 14 percent. By 2018, natural gas supplied 35.2 percent of the nation's electricity and coal only 27.5 percent. Consequently, employment in the coal industry fell by about 27 percent from 2005 to 2015. These numbers showed a slight uptick in 2016–2019 under the Trump administration, driven primarily by an increase in demand for coal exports, but the gains were small (still below 2015 levels) and were not expected to last. Forecasts of coal's continued decline have led many to call for a concerted effort to help coal-mining communities make a just transition to a new economic model. Such a transition will require commitment and creativity on the part of both public and private entities at all levels. As Helen Lewis wrote more than twenty years ago: "It is time to be creative, dream new dreams, develop new models. Let us plan for resurrection, not designate the region as a further sacrifice area."[48]

Education

In terms of educational attainment, the Appalachian region has achieved near parity with the nation in high school graduation rates, but it still lags in postsecondary graduation rates. In 1960, 32 percent of the Appalachian population had completed high school, compared with 42 percent of the US population. Only 5 percent of Appalachian residents had earned a college degree, compared with nearly 8 percent of all Americans. In 2017, 86.4 percent of adults in Appalachia had earned at least a high school diploma, nearly equal to the national average of 87.3 percent. But despite the region's dramatic progress in the percentage of residents completing at least a bachelor's degree (23.7 percent), it was still well behind the national average (30.9 percent).[49]

Technology

Access to technology and the internet is increasingly vital for education, economic opportunities, and health care. The Appalachian region has made progress in this area but still trails the rest of the nation. In 2017, 82.2 percent of Appalachian households had access to a computer device, while the national average was 87.2 percent. The results were similar for broadband internet access: 72.3 percent of Appalachian households had a broadband subscription, compared with 78.1 percent nationally. Like so many measures, these numbers vary widely across the region. For example, broadband access is highest in metropolitan areas and in Northern Appalachia, and it is lowest in Central Appalachia and in the most rural counties.[50]

Environment

While Appalachia is home to some of the most stunning examples of wilderness and natural resources in the eastern United States, it has also seen environmental devastation on a massive scale. Stricter regulations and increased conservation efforts in recent decades have slowed environmental impacts in many respects, but the region continues to face major threats in the twenty-first century. Few realize that the rupture of a containment dike at the TVA Kingston coal ash spill in Roane County, Tennessee, in 2008 released 1.1 billion gallons of coal ash slurry—the worst disaster of its kind in US history. The volume was six times that of the 2010 BP *Deepwater Horizon* oil spill in the Gulf of Mexico and 100 times the volume of the 1989 *Exxon Valdez* oil spill. In 2014 a leaky tank released up to 10,000 gallons of toxic chemicals into the Elk River in West Virginia, affecting the drinking water of more than 300,000 people in nine counties.[51]

But perhaps the greatest threat to the environment in recent decades is the practice of "mountaintop-removal" coal mining, a particularly egregious form of surface mining in which the tops of the mountains are removed by explosives and machinery to reveal coal seams, while the resulting tons of waste rock fill the valleys below. This process has devastated the Appalachian Mountains on a massive scale. Through 2015 about 1.5 million acres of Central Appalachia, 7.1 percent of the land area, had been surface mined—an area 18 percent larger than the state of Delaware. At least 1,000 mountains have been destroyed forever, and more than 2,000 miles of streams have been buried under the waste. In addition to irretrievably scarring the landscape and obliterating wildlife habitat, this practice has terrible effects on the watershed. The water supplies of thousands of residents who live near or downstream of mountaintop-removal sites have been contaminated, causing long-term health effects.[52] As this volume explores, environmental factors are one reason that the health and well-being of the Appalachian population have improved since the 1960s but remain well below the rest of the nation in many respects. This is the subject of much of the rest of this book.

Paradox, Promise, and Perspective

As this survey has shown, the history of Appalachia is a chronicle of enduring contrasts. Noted Appalachian writer Wilma Dykeman reflected on this curious fact in her influential 1955 book on the history of one of the great Appalachian rivers: "The French Broad [River] country, like most of the mountain region which surrounds it, nourishes paradox. That is the source of much of its allure—and despair. The roots of the paradoxes, the problems, the promises, run deep into the past. This is one glimpse into that past, and one glance at the present. Perhaps it provides some perspective for the future."[53] More than six decades later, Dykeman's words are still appropriate. Twenty-first-century Appalachia remains a region of paradox and promise—a place of abundant resources, rich history, natural and cultural diversity, and enduring tradition arrayed against a legacy of misunderstanding, exploitation, and stereotyping. And yet, alongside these apparent paradoxes, the region holds tremendous promise for its people and for the rest of the nation. Appalachia's story is both a cautionary tale, admonishing us not to repeat the mistakes of the past, and an inspiring fable, reminding us what is truly important in our relationships with one another and with the natural world. This perspective is badly needed as the region, the nation, and the world seek equitable solutions to the many challenges facing humanity today.

Notes

Epigraph: Richard Straw, "Appalachian History," in *A Handbook to Appalachia,* ed. Grace Toney Edwards, JoAnn Aust Asbury, and Ricky L. Cox (Knoxville: University of Tennessee Press, 2006), 1–26.

1. Olive Dame Campbell, *The Life and Works of John C. Campbell,* ed. Elizabeth McCutcheon (Lexington: University Press of Kentucky, 2016), 118; John C. Campbell, *The Southern Highlander and His Homeland* (1921; reprint, Lexington: University Press of Kentucky, 1969), xxi, 8–9. Olive Dame Campbell was a pioneer in studying the ballad tradition in Appalachia and was instrumental in bringing British ballad collector Cecil Sharp to the mountains, with whom she authored *English Folk Songs from the Southern Appalachians* (1917). In 1925 Olive founded the John C. Campbell Folk School in Brasstown, North Carolina. See also Olive Dame Campbell and Elizabeth M. Williams, *Appalachian Travels: The Diary of Olive Dame Campbell* (Lexington: University Press of Kentucky, 2012).

2. Ron Eller, "Appalachia in the Era of Trump: Uneven Ground Revisited" (lecture, University of Kentucky, Lexington, September 28, 2017); Jeff Biggers, *The United States of Appalachia: How Southern Mountaineers Brought Independence, Culture, and Enlightenment to America* (Emeryville, CA: Shoemaker and Hoard, 2006), xii–xiii.

3. David Walls, "On the Naming of Appalachia," in *An Appalachian Symposium: Essays Written in Honor of Cratis D. Williams,* ed. J. W. Williamson (Boone, NC: Appalachian State University Press, 1977), 56–76.

4. S. H. B. Clark, *Geology of the Southern Appalachian Mountains: U.S. Geological Survey Scientific Investigations Map 2830* (Washington, DC: US Geological Survey, 2008), https://pubs.usgs.gov/sim/2830/; Don W. Byerly and John J. Reston, "Geology," in *Encyclopedia of Appalachia,* ed. Rudy Abramson and Jean Haskell (Knoxville: University of Tennessee Press, 2006), 3–7.

5. Charlotte Muir, "Biodiversity of the Southern Appalachians," Highlands Biological Station, Western Carolina University, https://highlandsbiological.org/biodiversity-of-the-southern-appalachians/; Donald Davis, *Where There Are Mountains: An Environmental History of the Southern Appalachians* (Athens: University of Georgia Press, 2000).

6. William Bartram, *Travels through North and South Carolina, Georgia, East and West Florida, the Cherokee Country, the Extensive Territories of the Muscogulges, or Creek Confederacy, and the Country of the Chactaws; Containing an Account of the Soil and Natural Productions of Those Regions, Together with Observations on the Manners of the Indians* (Philadelphia: James Johnston, 1791), 352; "Documenting the American South," University of North Carolina Academic Library, https://docsouth.unc.edu/nc/bartram/bartram.html.

7. Stewart Scales, Emily Satterwhite, and Abby August, "Berea by Frost and Hayes 1896," Mapping Appalachia: A Digital Collection, https://mapappalachia.geography.vt.edu /about/berea/; Campbell, *Southern Highlander,* 10–17.

8. Appalachian Regional Commission, *The Appalachian Region* (Washington, DC: ARC, 2020), https://www.arc.gov/appalachian_region/TheAppalachianRegion.asp.

9. Richard A. Straw, introduction to *High Mountains Rising: Appalachia in Time and Place,* ed. Richard A. Straw and H. Tyler Blethen (Urbana: Southern Illinois University Press, 2004), 1–6; John Alexander Williams, *Appalachia: A History* (Chapel Hill: University of North Carolina Press, 2002), 13–14; John Alexander Williams, "Counting Yesterday's People: Using Aggregate Data to Address the Problem of Appalachia's Boundaries," *Journal of Appalachian Studies* 2, no. 1 (Spring 1996): 3–27. Williams used six definitions of Appalachia: Frost-Berea (1901), Campbell (1921), US Department of Agriculture (1935), Ford (1962), ARC (1965), and Raitz and Ulack (1984). These definitions of the region varied from 190 counties (Ford) to 445 counties (Raitz and Ulack). Scholars at Virginia Tech have developed an excellent website detailing the many historical attempts to map Appalachia; see Stewart Scales, Emily Satterwhite, and Abigail August, Mapping Appalachia: A Digital Collection, May 2018, https:// www.mapappalachia.geography.vt.edu/. See also Stewart Scales, Emily Satterwhite, and Abigail August, "Mapping Appalachia's Boundaries: Historiographic Overview and Digital Collection," *Journal of Appalachian Studies* 24, no. 1 (Spring 2018): 89–100.

10. "Alleghania, Alleghania, God Shed His Grace on Thee. . .," *American Heritage* 30, no. 5 (1979), https://www.americanheritage.com/alleghania-alleghania-god-shed-his-grace-thee; Edgar Allan Poe, "The Name of the Nation," *Graham's Magazine,* December 1846, in *The Portable Edgar Allan Poe,* ed. J. Gerald Kennedy (New York: Penguin, 2006), 600.

11. Charles Hudson, *Knights of Spain, Warriors of the Sun: Hernando de Soto and the South's Ancient Chiefdoms* (Athens: University of Georgia Press, 1997); Charles Hudson, *The Forgotten Centuries: Indians and Europeans in the American South, 1521–1704* (Athens: University of Georgia Press, 1994), 251–72.

12. James Mooney, *History, Myths, and Sacred Formulas of the Cherokee, 1891 and 1900* (Fairview, NC: Historical Images, 1992), 14; C. Clifford Boyd Jr., "Native Americans," in Straw and Blethen, *High Mountains Rising,*7–16; Theda Perdue and Michael D. Green, *The Cherokee Nation and the Trail of Tears* (New York: Penguin, 2008), 6.

13. Boyd, "Native Americans," 7–16; John Ehle, *Trail of Tears: The Rise and Fall of the Cherokee Nation* (New York: Random House, 1988); Perdue and Green, *Cherokee Nation*; Charles Hudson, *The Southeastern Indians* (Knoxville: University of Tennessee Press, 1976), 455–65.

14. William H. Turner, introduction to *Blacks in Appalachia,* ed. William H. Turner and Edward J. Cabbell (Lexington: University Press of Kentucky, 1985), xvii–xxiii, xix.

15. James G. Leyburn, *The Scotch-Irish: A Social History* (Chapel Hill: University of North Carolina Press, 1962); H. Tyler Blethen and Curtis W. Wood Jr., *From Ulster to Carolina: The Migration of the Scotch-Irish to Southwestern North Carolina* (Raleigh: North Carolina Department of Cultural Resources, 1998).

16. H. Tyler Blethen, "Pioneer Settlement," in Straw and Blethen, *High Mountains Rising,* 17–29.

17. Steven Stoll, *Ramp Hollow: The Ordeal of Appalachia* (New York: Hill and Wang, 2017), xiv; J. Todd Nesbitt, "Economic Distributism in Appalachia," *Journal of Appalachian Studies* 25, no. 1 (Spring 2019): 26–48; Ronald D. Eller, "Land as Commodity: Industrialization of the Appalachian Forests, 1880–1940," in *The Great Forest: An Appalachian Story,* ed. Barry M. Buxton and Malinda L. Crutchfield (Boone, NC: Appalachian Consortium, 1985), 28, https://www.jstor.org/stable/j.ctt1xp3n09.6.

18. Paul Salstrom, *Appalachia's Path to Dependency: Rethinking a Region's Economic History, 1730–1940* (Lexington: University Press of Kentucky, 1994), xiii; James N. Gregory, *The Southern Diaspora: How the Great Migrations of Black and White Southerners Transformed America* (Chapel Hill: University of North Carolina Press, 2005).

19. Eller, "Land as Commodity," 40; US National Park Service, "Quick History of the National Park Service," 2018, https://www.nps.gov/articles/quick-nps-history.htm; Appalachian Trail Conservancy, "The Appalachian Trail," 2020, https://www.appalachiantrail.org/our-work/about-us/.

20. John Cheves and Bill Estep, "Chapter 3: The World Comes to Whitesburg to Take Harry Caudill's 'Poverty Tour,'" *Lexington Herald-Leader,* December 19, 2012, https://www.kentucky.com/news/special-reports/fifty-years-of-night/article44393733.html.

21. Appalachian Regional Commission, Center for Regional Economic Competitiveness, and West Virginia University, *Appalachia Then and Now: Examining Changes to the Appalachian Region since 1965* (Washington, DC: ARC, 2015); Jeremy Richardson, "Despite Rhetoric, Coal Jobs Not Set to Increase in the Future," Union of Concerned Scientists, January 26, 2018, https://blog.ucsusa.org/jeremy-richardson/despite-rhetoric-coal-jobs-not-set-to-increase-in-the-future.

22. William Goodell Frost, "Our Contemporary Ancestors in the Southern Mountains," *Atlantic,* March 1899, https://www.theatlantic.com/magazine/toc/1899/03/.

23. Arnold J. Toynbee, *A Study of History,* abridged by D. G. Somervell (Oxford: Oxford University Press, 1946), 464; Jack E. Weller, *Yesterday's People: Life in Contemporary Appalachia* (Lexington: University Press of Kentucky, 1965); Bruce Roberts and Nancy Roberts, *Where Time Stood Still: A Portrait of Appalachia* (New York: Collier-MacMillan, 1970), 1.

24. Ann Toplovich, "Native American Trails," in *Tennessee Encyclopedia,* 2017, http://tennesseeencyclopedia.net/entries/native-american-trails/; William E. Myer, *Indian Trails of the Southeast* (Washington, DC: US Bureau of American Ethnology, 1928); Ronald L. Lewis, "Beyond Isolation and Homogeneity," in *Back Talk from Appalachia: Confronting Stereotypes* (Lexington: University Press of Kentucky, 2007), 21–43; David S. Hsiung, *Two Worlds in the Tennessee Mountains: Exploring the Origins of Appalachian Stereotypes* (Lexington: University Press of Kentucky, 2007), 8–17.

25. Biggers, *United States of Appalachia,* xv.

26. Michael Montgomery, "In the Appalachians They Speak Like Shakespeare," in *Language Myths,* ed. Laurie Bauer and Peter Trudgill (London: Penguin, 1999), 66–76; Jennifer Cramer, "Is Shakespeare Still in the Holler? The Death of a Language Myth," *Southern Journal of Linguistics* 38, no. 1 (2014): 195–207, https://uknowledge.uky.edu/lin_facpub/70; "The History of Appalachian English: Why We Talk Differently," *Appalachian Magazine,* November 23, 2017, http://appalachianmagazine.com/2017/11/23/the-history-of-appalachian-english-why-we-talk-differently/. Proponents of this myth sometimes claim that Appalachians speak the language of Chaucer, who predated the Elizabethan age by more than 150 years.

27. Blethen, "Pioneer Settlement," 19; William H. Turner, "The Demography of Black Appalachia: Past and Present," in Turner and Cabbell, *Blacks in Appalachia,* 237–61; Kelvin Pollard and Linda A. Jacobsen, *The Appalachian Region: A Data Overview from the 2013–2017 American Community Survey* (Washington, DC: ARC, 2019), https://www.arc.gov/research/researchreportdetails.asp?REPORT_ID=159; Ronald L. Lewis, *Welsh Americans: A History of Assimilation in the Coalfields* (Chapel Hill: University of North Carolina Press, 2008); Heidi Taylor-Caudill and Whitney Hays, "Immigrants in the Coalfields," University of Kentucky Special Collections, http://iia.uky.edu/immigrantsinthecoalfields; Stevan R. Jackson, "Peoples of Appalachia: Cultural Diversity within the Mountain Region," in *A Handbook to Appalachia,* ed. Grace Toney Edwards, JoAnn Aust Asbury, and Ricky L. Cox (Knoxville: University of Tennessee Press, 2006), 31.

28. Mario Luis Small, David J. Harding, and Michele Lamont, "Reconsidering Culture and Poverty," *Annals of the American Academy of Political and Social Science* 629 (May 2010): 6–27; Dwight B. Billings and Kathleen M. Blee, *The Road to Poverty: The Making of Wealth and Hardship in Appalachia* (Cambridge: Cambridge University Press, 2000), 13.

29. J. D. Vance, *Hillbilly Elegy: A Memoir of a Family and Culture in Crisis* (New York: HarperCollins, 2016); Anthony Harkins and Meredith McCarroll, eds., *Appalachian Reckoning: A Region Responds to Hillbilly Elegy* (Morgantown: West Virginia University Press, 2019).

30. Richard E. Nisbett and Dov Cohen, *Culture of Honor: The Psychology of Violence in the South* (Boulder, CO: Westview Press, 1996); Nigel Barber, "Is Southern Violence Due to a Culture of Honor? Did Scots-Irish Settlers Transmit Violent Tendencies to the South?" *Psychology Today,* April 2, 2009, https://www.psychologytoday.com/us/blog/the-human-beast/200904/is-southern-violence-due-culture-honor.

31. Altina Waller, *Feud: Hatfields, McCoys, and Social Change in Appalachia* (Chapel Hill: University of North Carolina Press, 1988); "Hatfield McCoy Feud & Trails," Hatfield-McCoy Regional Recreation Authority," 2018–2020, https://trailsheaven.com/about-the-trails/hatfield-mccoy-feud-trails/.

32. Biggers, *United States of Appalachia,* xii–xiii.

33. Joshua Aronson, Diana Burgess, Sean M. Phelan, and Lindsay Juarez, "Unhealthy Interactions: The Role of Stereotype Threat in Health Disparities," *American Journal of Public Health* 103, no. 1 (January 2013): 50–56; Diana J. Burgess et al., "Stereotype Threat and Health Disparities: What Medical Educators and Future Physicians Need to Know," *Journal of General Internal Medicine* 25, suppl. 2 (2010): 169–77; Claude M. Steele, *Whistling Vivaldi: How Stereotypes Affect Us and What We Can Do* (New York: Norton, 2011). Studies on the effects of stereotyping in Appalachia include Angela K. Cooke-Jackson and Elizabeth K. Hansen, "Appalachian Culture and Reality TV: The Ethical Dilemma of Stereotyping Others," *Journal of Mass Media Ethics* 23, no. 3 (2008): 183–200; George Towers, "West Virginia's Lost Youth: Appalachian Stereotypes and Residential Preferences," *Journal of Geography* 104, no. 2 (2005): 74–84; Kirk Hazen and Sarah Hamilton, "A Dialect Turned Inside Out: Migration and the Appalachian Diaspora," *Journal of English Linguistics* 36, no. 2 (June 2008): 105–28.

34. Clifford Geertz, *The Interpretation of Cultures* (New York: Basic Books, 1973); Akhil Gupta and James Ferguson, *Culture, Power, Place: Explorations in Critical Anthropology* (Durham, NC: Duke University Press, 1997).

35. Douglas Reichert Powell, *Critical Regionalism: Connecting Politics and Culture in the American Landscape* (Chapel Hill: University of North Carolina Press, 2007), 4–22.

36. Edward S. Casey, "How to Get from Space to Place," in *Senses of Place,* ed. Steven Feld and Keith H. Basso (Santa Fe, NM: School of American Research Press, 1996), 13–52.

37. Esther M. Sternberg, *Healing Places: The Science of Place and Well-Being* (Cambridge, MA: Harvard University Press, 2009), 1–2, 10.

38. Edmund Burke, *A Philosophical Enquiry into the Origin of Our Ideas of the Sublime and Beautiful* (1757; reprint, Oxford: Oxford University Press, 1998), 66; Robert MacFarlane, *Mountains of the Mind: Adventures in Reaching the Summit* (New York: Random House, 2004), chap. 1, loc. 319–20, 335–36, Kindle.

39. Susan E. Keefe, introduction to *Appalachian Cultural Competency: A Guide for Medical, Mental Health, and Social Service Professionals,* ed. Susan E. Keefe (Knoxville: University of Tennessee Press, 2005), 10–14.

40. Keefe, introduction to *Appalachian Cultural Competency,* 10–14.

41. Keefe, introduction to *Appalachian Cultural Competency,* 3. I prefer the term *intercultural competence* because it implies ongoing interaction and dialogue between cultures rather than a one-way process. Although intercultural competence is a fairly recent concept in some disciplines, communication studies scholars have done extensive research on intercultural communication over many years, providing foundational principles that underlie much of the recent work in the area.

42. US Department of Health and Human Services, Office of Minority Health, "National Culturally and Linguistically Appropriate Services Standards," https://thinkculturalhealth .hhs.gov/clas/standards; US Department of Health and Human Services, Office of Minority Health, "Tracking CLAS," https://thinkculturalhealth.hhs.gov/clas/clas-tracking-map.

43. ARC, *Appalachia Then and Now.*

44. Pollard and Jacobsen, *Appalachian Region.*

45. Pollard and Jacobsen, *Appalachian Region.*

46. ARC, *Appalachia Then and Now;* Appalachian Regional Commission, *Relative Poverty Rates in Appalachia, 2013–2017* (Washington, DC: ARC, 2018); Appalachian Regional Commission, *ARC-Designated Distressed Counties, Fiscal Year 2019* (Washington, DC: ARC, 2019); Pollard and Jacobsen, *Appalachian Region.*

47. ARC, *Appalachia Then and Now;* Appalachian Regional Commission, *Relative Unemployment Rates in Appalachia, 2017* (Washington, DC: ARC, 2018).

48. ARC, *Appalachia Then and Now;* ARC, *Relative Unemployment Rates in Appalachia, 2017;* Eric Bowen et al., *An Overview of the Coal Economy in Appalachia* (Chicago: Walsh Center for Rural Health Analysis at the University of Chicago and ARC, 2017); US Energy Information Administration, *What Is US Electricity Generation by Energy Source?* (Washington, DC: USEIA, 2019); Tom DiChristopher, "Coal-Mining Jobs Are Holding Steady under Trump's Watch—That Could Become Harder This Year," CNBC.com, March 8, 2010, https://www .cnbc.com/2019/03/08/coal-mining-jobs-are-holding-steady-under-trumps-watch.html; Helen Matthews Lewis, "Coal and after Coal," in *Living Social Justice in Appalachia,* ed. Patricia D. Beaver and Judith Jennings (Lexington: University Press of Kentucky, 2012), 135–38.

49. ARC, *Appalachia Then and Now;* Appalachian Regional Commission, *High School and College Completion Rates in Appalachia, 2017* (Washington, DC: ARC, 2018).

50. Pollard and Jacobsen, *Appalachian Region.*

51. US Environmental Protection Agency, *TVA Kingston Site Case Study* (Washington, DC: EPA, 2017), https://www.epa.gov/remedytech/tva-kingston-site-case-study-0; US Environmental Protection Agency, *Deepwater Horizon: BP Gulf of Mexico Oil Spill* (Washington, DC: EPA, 2017), https://www.epa.gov/enforcement/deepwater-horizon-bp-gulf-mexico

-oil-spill; US Environmental Protection Agency, *Exxon Valdez Spill Profile* (Washington, DC: EPA, 2017), https://www.epa.gov/emergency-response/exxon-valdez-spill-profile; US Chemical Safety and Hazard Investigation Board, *Investigation Report: Chemical Spill Contaminates Public Water Supply in Charleston, West Virginia* (Washington, DC: CSHIB, 2014).

52. Andrew A. Pericak et al., "Mapping the Yearly Extent of Surface Coal Mining in Central Appalachia Using Landsat and Google Earth Engine," *Public Library of Science* 13, no. 7 (July 25, 2018), https://www.ncbi.nlm.nih.gov/pmc/articles/PMC6059389/.

53. Wilma Dykeman, *The French Broad* (New York: Henry Holt, 1955; reprint, Newport, TN: Wakestone Books, 1999), vii.

3

Appalachian Health

An Overview of Mortality and Morbidity

JULIE MARSHALL AND LOGAN THOMAS

A healthy population is a critical component of a vibrant, thriving community. The overall well-being of a community reflects almost every issue impacting that community, especially its current economic conditions and its future economic prospects. Good health and a strong economy move in tandem. In Appalachia, poor health statistics parallel poor economic conditions. They are both a contributor to and a by-product of socioeconomic conditions. Appalachia's higher poverty rate (relative to the rest of the nation), lower household income, and lower levels of educational attainment influence—and are influenced by—its lower life expectancy, higher infant mortality rate, and higher rates of diseases such as diabetes and obesity.[1]

Providing a comprehensive overview of the health and well-being of the people of Appalachia is an important, foundational step toward better understanding the overall challenges facing the region. Measuring a population's health, documenting health disparities between Appalachia and the rest of the United States, and working to reduce those disparities are critical elements of any plan to create a successful future for Appalachia.

To assess the current health landscape across Appalachia, this chapter examines the region's performance on fifteen measures of health status relative to that of the rest of the country. To aid in characterizing the region's health, the fifteen indicators are grouped into two broad categories: mortality and morbidity. These categories were chosen to reflect the current and prospective health of the population. Other chapters address other important components of population health, including access to health care, risk factors, and social determinants of health. Together, the indicators explored in this book provide an overview of health in Appalachia and include both health outcomes—such as specific measures of mortality and morbidity—and the factors that drive or influence health outcomes—such as smoking prevalence, physical inactivity, and the supply of health care providers, among others.[2]

To provide a more nuanced view of how the region performed on these fifteen indicators, the county-level data examined in each category are shown in groupings based on *national* quintiles—five levels of performance created from the distribution of values across every county in the United States. Accordingly, if the Appalachian region's county distribution matched the national distribution, each quintile would contain eighty-four counties (20 percent of the 420 counties in Appalachia). Reporting the data using the framework of national quintiles provides insight into how Appalachia's county-level health outcomes are distributed among performance levels, and it indicates how Appalachia compares with the rest of the nation. This chapter also compares outcomes between the region's metropolitan (metro) and rural counties and among Appalachia's five subregions. Just as there is a distinct difference in the experiences of residents in metro and rural counties, disparities also exist in Appalachia's subregions.[3]

The findings discussed here identify numerous issues that need to be addressed to improve the health status of the region. However, along with these challenges come opportunities to adopt strategies and implement evidence-based interventions to improve the health of the nearly 26 million people who call Appalachia home.

Category 1: Mortality

Understanding the major causes of death in a population is key not only to determining its current health status but also to gaining insight into the types of interventions that will be most effective in improving health outcomes. The ten mortality measures included here examine rates of death due to eight specific causes, as well as infant mortality rates and a broad measure of premature mortality:

- Heart disease
- Cancer
- Chronic obstructive pulmonary disease (COPD)
- Injury
- Poisoning
- Stroke
- Diabetes
- Suicide
- Infant mortality
- Years of potential life lost (YPLL)

The age-adjusted rate for each indicator examined was higher (worse) in the Appalachian region than in the non-Appalachian United States (table 3.1). In fact, the rates in Appalachia were all at least 10 percent higher than the rates in

Table 3.1. Mortality Indicators for Appalachia and the Non-Appalachian United States

Indicator	Appalachian Region	Non-Appalachian US
Heart disease mortality rate per 100,000 population, 2008–2014	204.1	173.0
Cancer mortality rate per 100,000 population, 2008–2014	184.0	166.7
Injury mortality rate (including poisoning) per 100,000 population, 2008–2014	52.4	38.3
Poisoning mortality rate per 100,000 population, 2008–2014	20.4	14.4
COPD mortality rate per 100,000 population, 2008–2014	53.5	40.9
Stroke mortality rate per 100,000 population, 2008–2014	43.8	38.0
Diabetes mortality rate per 100,000 population, 2008–2014	23.8	21.3
Suicide mortality rate per 100,000 population, 2008–2014	14.5	12.2
Infant mortality rate per 1,000 live births, 2008–2014	7.1	6.1
Years of potential life lost, 2011–2013	8,291	6,515

Source: Julie L. Marshall et al., *Health Disparities in Appalachia* (Washington, DC: ARC, 2017).

the rest of the country, and for causes such as COPD and poisoning, the disparities were even greater.

Heart disease was the leading cause of death for adults in the United States in 2017, accounting for 23 percent of all deaths. The heart disease mortality rate in 2008–2014 was 18 percent higher in Appalachia than in the non-Appalachian United States. The risk factors for heart disease include a number of behaviors and conditions, such as smoking, obesity, diabetes, excessive alcohol use, physical inactivity, hypertension, high cholesterol, and an unhealthy diet. Several of these risk factors are discussed in other chapters. Although the risk for heart disease can be influenced by immutable factors such as age, race, and genetics, many of the other risk factors can be addressed. Reducing or improving these risk factors and behaviors may decrease mortality from a number of causes, not just heart disease.[4]

Cancer was the second leading cause of death in the United States in 2017, and a recent study found that in a number of states, cancer has surpassed heart disease as the leading cause of death. The cancer mortality rate in the

Appalachian region in 2008–2014 was 10 percent higher than in the rest of the country. Not all cancers can be prevented, but the risk of getting cancer can be reduced by making healthy lifestyle choices, including avoiding smoking and exposure to secondhand smoke, protecting skin from ultraviolet rays, limiting alcohol consumption, and maintaining a healthy body weight. The Centers for Disease Control and Prevention (CDC) recommends regular screenings for breast, cervical, colorectal, and lung cancers, as early detection allows earlier treatment and a better chance of survival.

Unintentional injury became the third leading cause of death in the United States in 2016, surpassing deaths due to chronic lower respiratory disease. The mortality rate due to injury was 37 percent higher in Appalachia than in the non-Appalachian United States in 2008–2014. Mortality from injury includes deaths due to unintentional injuries and accidents such as motor vehicle crashes, falls, and poisoning. Poisoning includes deaths associated with pharmaceutical and illicit drug abuse and overdose; although the ingestion of other chemicals also falls under this category, these incidents are relatively rare. A recent study noted that deaths due to drug poisoning are the leading cause of injury-related death and have outnumbered deaths due to firearms, motor vehicle crashes, suicide, and homicide since 2011. Deaths due to poisoning were 42 percent higher in the Appalachian region than in the rest of the country in 2008–2014.[5]

Recent research has shown that in 2015 there were 5,594 deaths among those aged fifteen to sixty-four in Appalachia due to drug overdose, and 69 percent of these deaths were caused by opioids (opium, heroin, methadone, other opioids, and synthetic narcotics). This research also explored mortality in Appalachia due to "diseases of despair"—drug overdose, suicide, and alcoholic liver disease—and found that in 2017 the combined mortality rate was 45 percent higher in Appalachia than in the rest of the United States. Several factors contribute to higher rates of opioid misuse and overdose deaths in Appalachia. According to a 2019 report published by the Appalachian Regional Commission (ARC), higher rates of injury-prone employment, aggressive marketing of prescription pain medications to physicians, and an insufficient supply of behavioral and public health services targeting opioid misuse contribute to the higher rates of opioid misuse and mortality in Appalachia. The report's authors state that these factors, combined with high poverty rates throughout the region, create a multifaceted public health threat. They go on to recommend that "equally multifaceted intervention strategies are needed to address opioid misuse and overdose deaths in Appalachia."[6]

Chronic lower respiratory disease, including COPD, was the fourth leading cause of death in the United States in 2017. Over the 2008–2014 period, deaths due to COPD were 31 percent higher in Appalachia than in the rest of the country. Smoking is the most significant risk factor for COPD, and areas with higher rates of smoking tend to have higher mortality rates from COPD. Other risk factors for COPD include genetic factors, respiratory infections, and environmental conditions such as poor air quality. Recent studies have explored the relationship between respiratory diseases and exposure to coal dust. One study found that cumulative lifetime exposure to coal dust increased the risk of death from COPD, and another study found that coal dust caused a number of lung and respiratory diseases, including COPD. A 2009 study found that cumulative exposure to coal dust was a significant predictor of emphysema, even after controlling for other factors such as age, race, and cigarette smoking.[7]

Cerebrovascular disease, or stroke, was the fifth leading cause of death in the United States in 2017. The mortality rate due to stroke was 15 percent higher in Appalachia than in the non-Appalachian United States in 2008–2014. Risk factors for stroke fall into three broad categories: underlying health conditions, lifestyle choices, and genetics. Underlying health conditions that may increase the risk of stroke include a previous stroke or mini-stroke, high blood pressure, high cholesterol, heart disease, diabetes, and sickle cell disease. An unhealthy diet, physical inactivity, obesity, excessive alcohol intake, and tobacco use are all lifestyle factors that increase the risk of stroke. Although there are a number of preventable risk factors for stroke, others, such as heredity, age, gender, and ethnicity, cannot be changed. Access to quick treatment after a stroke is critical for reducing stroke mortality and disability. Treatment with tissue plasminogen activator (tPA) within four to five hours after a stoke significantly improves the odds of a good outcome; earlier treatment has been associated with larger proportional benefits. Although the number of deaths due to stroke has generally declined over the last forty years, this downward trend has recently slowed among black Americans and reversed among Hispanics.[8]

Diabetes was the seventh leading cause of death in the United States in 2017. During the 2008–2014 period, the diabetes mortality rate was 12 percent higher in Appalachia than in the rest of the country. Despite the prevalence of diabetes, one study found that only 39 percent of death certificates for diabetics noted that they had the disease, and only 10 percent listed diabetes as the underlying cause of death. The relationship between mortality and diabetes is not always clear, whereas with many other diseases, such as cancer, the links are more direct and easier to measure. It is therefore likely that diabetes mortality rates are underreported, as physicians often cite one of the disease's complications—heart attack, stroke, or kidney failure—as the primary cause of death, without mentioning diabetes. In addition to having a higher risk of premature death, people with diabetes have higher rates of comorbid conditions such as heart disease, kidney disease, kidney failure, neuropathy, poor digestion, and issues related to vision, oral health, and mental health.[9]

Suicide was the tenth leading cause of death in the United States in 2017. The mortality rate due to suicide was 19 percent higher in Appalachia than in the non-Appalachian United States in 2008–2014. Risk factors for suicide include a family history of suicide, previous suicide attempts, a history of mental health disorders such as depression, a history of alcohol and substance abuse, feelings of hopelessness, local epidemics of suicide, isolation, lack of access to mental health care providers, and physical illness. Individuals who are opioid dependent are at increased risk of suicide, suggesting that as the epidemic of opioid misuse and dependence is addressed, those in recovery must be monitored for suicide risk and provided with appropriate mental health care and other resources.[10]

In 2016 firearms were the leading mechanism of suicide for males older than fifteen in the United States, and recent work has identified suicide as a major component of "deaths of despair," a leading driver of increased mortality among middle-aged white males. In fact, the number of suicides in the United States has increased each year since 2003. Rural areas have higher rates of suicide across both genders and all age groups, and the overall disparity between rural and urban suicide rates is growing, particularly among persons aged ten to twenty-four.[11]

Infant mortality is a commonly used health indicator. Previous studies have shown that the factors influencing infant mortality, such as socioeconomic well-being, environmental quality, and access to health care, also impact the overall health status of the population. During the 2008–2014 period, the infant mortality rate in Appalachia was 16 percent higher than the rate in the non-Appalachian United States. A number of factors contribute to infant mortality, including preterm birth, low birth weight, birth defects, maternal pregnancy complications, sudden infant death syndrome (SIDS), and accidents. Many causes of infant death are preventable. Prenatal care can reduce prenatal injuries and preterm birth, both of which contribute to infant mortality. Unhealthy maternal behaviors such as smoking, drinking alcohol, and being physically inactive are also risk factors, so decreasing or eliminating these behaviors can reduce the risk of infant mortality. The incidence of SIDS, the leading cause of infant death outside the perinatal period, can be reduced by implementing healthy sleeping habits, reducing smoking in the home, and other interventions.[12]

Another widely used measure of the overall health of a community is the early death rate. Years of potential life lost (YPLL) measures the cumulative

Table 3.2. Mortality Indicators for Rural and Large Metro Counties

Indicator	Rural Counties	Large Metro Counties
Heart disease mortality rate per 100,000 population, 2008–2014	234	184
Cancer mortality rate per 100,000 population, 2008–2014	202	175
Injury mortality rate (including poisoning) per 100,000 population, 2008–2014	67.4	45.7
Poisoning mortality rate per 100,000 population, 2008–2014	26.2	18.7
COPD mortality rate per 100,000 population, 2008–2014	68.9	44.5
Stroke mortality rate per 100,000 population, 2008–2014	46.0	42.5
Diabetes mortality rate per 100,000 population, 2008–2014	27.7	20.3
Suicide mortality rate per 100,000 population, 2008–2014	15.9	13.1
Infant mortality rate per 1,000 live births, 2008–2014	8.0	6.7
Years of potential life lost, 2011–2013	10,100	7,221

Source: Julie L. Marshall et al., *Health Disparities in Appalachia* (Washington, DC: ARC, 2017).

number of years a population loses when people die before age seventy-five. During the 2011–2013 period, YPLL was 27 percent higher in Appalachia than in the rest of the country. The calculation of YPLL gives increased weight to deaths among younger populations because these deaths are more likely to be preventable and thus more responsive to interventions. YPLL is an important measure to consider when exploring ways to reduce mortality rates in a population.[13]

For all the mortality measures included in this section, Appalachia's rural counties had higher rates than the large metropolitan counties, signifying a stark rural-urban divide (table 3.2). Taken together, these disparities in mortality rates between rural and urban areas—within a region already facing disparities with the rest of the country—provide a comprehensive albeit grim overview of the health of the people living in Appalachia's rural communities.[14]

Stratifying the data by the five Appalachian subregions sheds light on the disparities in mortality indicators. For eight of the ten measures, the Central subregion performs the worst and has the highest mortality rates among the five subregions. The Southern subregion has the highest stroke mortality rate, and three subregions are tied for the highest infant mortality rate.[15]

Table 3.3. Distribution of Appalachian Counties among National Quintiles for Mortality Indicators

Indicator	Best Quintile		Second Best Quintile		Middle Quintile		Second Worst Quintile		Worst Quintile	
	No.	%	No.	%	No.	%	No.	%	No.	%
Heart disease deaths	15	4	56	13	76	18	115	27	158	38
Cancer deaths	29	7	49	12	83	20	101	24	158	38
COPD deaths	27	6	54	13	83	20	93	22	163	39
Injury deaths	28	7	59	14	80	19	106	25	147	35
Stroke deaths	40	10	69	16	90	21	111	26	110	26
Diabetes deaths	60	14	70	17	91	22	100	24	99	24
Poisoning deaths	24	6	31	7	56	13	114	27	195	46
Suicide deaths	46	11	69	16	108	26	127	30	70	17
Infant deaths	24	6	73	17	112	27	124	30	87	21
YPLL	13	3	63	15	81	19	105	25	156	37

Source: Julie L. Marshall et al., *Health Disparities in Appalachia* (Washington, DC: ARC, 2017).

Note: The number of counties may not sum to 420 due to missing or suppressed values.

The distribution of county-level mortality rates based on national quintiles provides another way to examine the disparities between Appalachia and the United States as a whole, as well as the disparities within the region (see table 3.3). Of the 420 counties in Appalachia, 163 counties (39 percent) had COPD mortality rates in the worst-performing national quintile, and only 27 counties (6 percent) were in the best-performing national quintile. There were 158 counties (38 percent) in the worst-performing national quintiles for both heart disease and cancer mortality. Only 13 counties (3 percent) were in the best-performing quintile for YPLL.

Compared with the rest of the United States, the Appalachian region performed poorly on each of the mortality measures included in this section. In other words, the people of Appalachia are dying from many of the same causes as people in the rest of the country, but at higher rates.

Category 2: Morbidity

Understanding the factors that impact quality of life is as important as understanding the factors that cause people to die. The health status of the people of Appalachia can be understood by examining five health measures:

- Physically unhealthy days
- Mentally unhealthy days

- HIV prevalence
- Diabetes prevalence
- Obesity prevalence

With the exception of HIV prevalence, each of these measures was higher (worse) in Appalachia than in the non-Appalachian United States (table 3.4).

"Physically unhealthy days" refers to the number of days per month the average adult aged eighteen years or older reports feeling physically unhealthy or in poor physical health. In 2014 the average Appalachian resident reported 4.1 physically unhealthy days per month, compared with 3.6 for the average adult living in the non-Appalachian United States. This measure is intended, in part, to examine overall quality of life—that is, how do people *feel* on a typical day? It is also intended to capture the aspects of poor health that may not be picked up by other measures that focus on specific diseases and illnesses.

Quantifying the number of days people feel sick or unhealthy is important when examining a community's health status. Physically unhealthy days can inhibit a person's ability to obtain gainful employment and, in some instances, can affect a person's mental health status. Past research has shown that physically unhealthy days are a precursor of future health issues and the need for medical care. In one analysis, counties with higher rates of physically unhealthy days also had higher unemployment and poverty rates, higher mortality rates, higher prevalence of disability, and lower rates of high school completion.[16]

Health is not solely about physical health—one's mental and emotional condition is just as critical to good health. "Mentally unhealthy days" refers to the number of days per month the average adult aged eighteen or older reports feeling mentally unhealthy or in poor mental health. In 2014 the average Appalachian resident reported 4.1 mentally unhealthy days per month, compared with 3.6 for the average adult living in the non-Appalachian United

Table 3.4. Morbidity Indicators for Appalachia and the Non-Appalachian United States

Indicator	Appalachian Region	Non-Appalachian US
Physically unhealthy days per month, 2014	4.1	3.6
Mentally unhealthy days per month, 2014	4.1	3.6
Adults with HIV per 100,000 population, 2013	153.5	373.1
Adult diabetes prevalence, 2012	11.9%	9.6%
Adult obesity prevalence, 2012	31.0%	27.1%

Source: Julie L. Marshall et al., *Health Disparities in Appalachia* (Washington, DC: ARC, 2017).

States. Counties whose residents report higher numbers of mentally unhealthy days have higher rates of unemployment, poverty, disability, and mortality, as well as lower high school completion rates. Higher levels of education and income are correlated with fewer mentally unhealthy days. Not every poor mental health day reflects a condition requiring treatment, as temporary conditions such as grief and stress are captured as part of this measure. Still, poor mental health days may influence a person's ability to work or to care for a dependent child or family member, and poor mental health may also lead to physical health issues.[17]

The HIV prevalence rate measures the number of people living with HIV per 100,000 population. HIV is a virus that attacks the immune system, making it difficult for the body to fight off infection and disease. More than 1.1 million people in the United States were living with HIV in 2016, and among those infected, it is estimated that one in seven had not been diagnosed. In 2013 the prevalence of HIV was 59 percent lower in Appalachia than in the non-Appalachian United States. In the United States, HIV is spread primarily through unprotected sex or the sharing of needles for injection drug use with someone who has HIV. There are a number of complications and conditions associated with HIV infection, including AIDS, certain cancers, tuberculosis, and hepatitis B and C. Because HIV and hepatitis B and C are transmitted through unprotected sexual contact or shared needles, people with HIV are at increased risk of hepatitis coinfection; in fact, CDC data show that approximately 75 percent of people with HIV who inject drugs also have hepatitis C. For hepatitis patients, HIV coinfection more than triples the risk for liver disease, liver failure, and liver-related death. A recent study identified counties vulnerable to the rapid spread of HIV through injection drug use, as well as those vulnerable to either developing or maintaining a high rate of hepatitis C infection. Of the 220 vulnerable counties identified nationwide, 64 percent (140 counties) were located in the Appalachian region.[18]

Diabetes prevalence is the percentage of adults aged twenty and older who have been diagnosed with type 1 or type 2 diabetes. In 2012 nearly 12 percent of Appalachian people had been diagnosed with diabetes, compared with 9.6 percent in the rest of the country. Type 2 diabetes is more common among adults than type 1; approximately 30 million adults have been diagnosed with type 2 diabetes in the United States. Unlike type 1 diabetes, type 2 diabetes is considered a preventable disease. According to the CDC, the risk factors for type 2 diabetes include older age, obesity, a family history of diabetes, a prior history of gestational diabetes, impaired glucose tolerance, physical inactivity, race, and ethnicity. Among the many possible complications of diabetes are blindness, kidney failure, neuropathy, and lower-extremity amputations. Diabetics have a lower quality of life and a higher risk of depression and premature death than those without diabetes. Diabetes prevalence has increased in conjunction with the rise in obesity and is much higher among rural residents than among those living in urban areas. Older individuals are at increased risk of developing diabetes, as are minorities and those who are physically inactive.[19]

Obesity prevalence is the percentage of adults aged eighteen and older who report height and weight measurements resulting in a body mass index of 30 or higher. Thirty-one percent of Appalachian individuals reported being obese in 2012, compared with 27.1 percent of residents in the non-Appalachian United States. The risk factors for obesity fall into three broad categories: behaviors, environmental factors, and genetics. Behaviors include eating patterns, physical activity levels, and medication use. Environmental factors include what types of food are accessible, marketing practices of the food industry, education and awareness, and whether the environment supports physical activity. Although the relationship between genetics and obesity is not entirely clear, differences in how people respond to both physical activity and certain foods suggest that genetics may play a role in obesity. Obesity increases the risk for a number of conditions such as high blood pressure, high cholesterol, type 2 diabetes, coronary heart disease, stroke, osteoarthritis, sleep apnea and other breathing problems, various cancers, poor quality of life, mental illness, and physical pain. There are well-known racial and socioeconomic patterns in obesity rates across the United States: the non-Hispanic black and Hispanic adult populations tend to have the highest rates, and both men and women with college degrees have a lower prevalence of obesity than those with less education.[20]

Like the previously discussed mortality measures, the rates for these morbidity measures tend to be higher in the Central Appalachia subregion than elsewhere in Appalachia. The Northern subregion has the lowest rates for four of the five measures.[21]

The distribution of these morbidity measures for all Appalachian counties, based on national quintiles, is shown in table 3.5. For mentally unhealthy days, 210 counties (50 percent) were in the worst-performing national quintile, and only 2 counties (less than 1 percent) were in the best-performing national quintile. Of the 420 counties in the region, 180 (43 percent) were in the worst-performing national quintile for diabetes prevalence, while only 12 counties (3 percent) were in the top-performing quintile. These results show that, with the exception of HIV prevalence, the health conditions analyzed were disproportionately worse throughout much of Appalachia than in the nation as a whole.

Residents of rural Appalachian counties had higher numbers of physically unhealthy days, higher numbers of mentally unhealthy days, greater diabetes

Table 3.5. Distribution of Appalachian Counties among National Quintiles for Morbidity Indicators

Indicator	Best Quintile		Second Best Quintile		Middle Quintile		Second Worst Quintile		Worst Quintile	
	No.	%	No.	%	No.	%	No.	%	No.	%
Physically unhealthy days	5	1	39	9	93	22	106	25	177	42
Mentally unhealthy days	2	0	19	5	96	23	93	22	210	50
HIV prevalence	89	21	109	26	104	25	61	15	20	5
Diabetes prevalence	12	3	32	8	68	16	128	30	180	43
Adult obesity prevalence	45	11	69	16	74	18	106	25	126	30

Source: Julie L. Marshall et al., *Health Disparities in Appalachia* (Washington, DC: ARC, 2017).

Note: The number of counties may not sum to 420 due to missing or suppressed values.

prevalence, and a greater prevalence of adult obesity than residents of the region's large metro counties. People living in rural counties reported 24 percent more physically unhealthy days than those living in large metro counties and 10 percent more mentally unhealthy days. Adult residents of rural Appalachian counties were also more likely to be obese than those living in large metro counties (33.1 versus 29.5 percent).[22]

Trends

Looking at changes in the performance of selected health indicators over time provides insight into how the health of Appalachian individuals has changed and how this compares with the change experienced in the rest of the country. The following discussion reviews changes in five measures of mortality between two time periods: 1989–1995 and 2008–2014. In this section, maps display county-level performance throughout the region for each of the periods, based on the counties' classification into national quintiles (figures 3.1–3.5). The analysis indicates that although improvements were made in each of these indicators, progress in Appalachia lagged behind that made in the rest of the United States.[23]

Indicator 1: YPLL

Between 1989–1995 and 2008–2014, the YPLL rate in Appalachia decreased by 8 percent, while the non-Appalachian United States experienced a much larger decline of 25 percent. Thus, despite the region's improvement, the gap between Appalachia and the rest of the nation increased between the two periods.

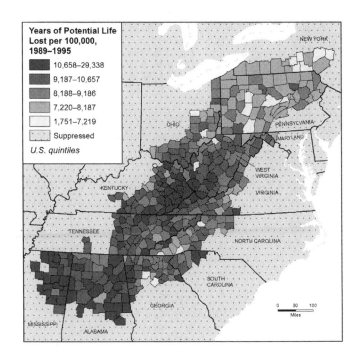

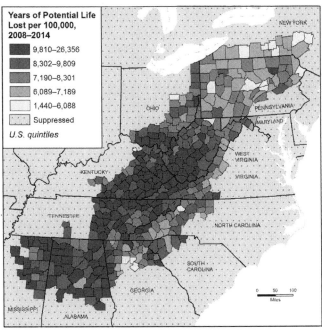

Figure 3.1. Years of potential life lost in the Appalachian region, 1989–1995 and 2008–2014. (*Source:* Julie L. Marshall et al., *Health Disparities in Appalachia* [Washington, DC: ARC, 2017])

During 1989–1995, the YPLL rate in Appalachia was 2 percent higher than that in the non-Appalachian United States; by 2008–2014, the YPLL rate in Appalachia was 25 percent higher than the non-Appalachian US rate, signifying a growing disparity.

Indicator 2: Cancer

Between 1989–1995 and 2008–2014, the cancer mortality rate in Appalachia decreased by 15 percent, versus a 21 percent decline in the rest of the country. Despite the region's improvement, the gap between Appalachia and the rest of the nation increased between the two periods. During 1989–1995, the cancer mortality rate in Appalachia was only 2 percent higher than the rate in the non-Appalachian United States; by 2008–2014, the rate in Appalachia was 10 percent higher than the non-Appalachian US rate, signifying a growing disparity.

Indicator 3: Heart Disease

Between 1989–1995 and 2008–2014, the heart disease mortality rate in Appalachia decreased by 39 percent, a slightly smaller improvement than the 43 percent decrease in the non-Appalachian United States. Despite the region's improvement, the gap between Appalachia and the rest of the country increased between the two periods. During 1989–1995, the heart disease mortality rate in Appalachia was 11 percent higher than in the rest of the country; by 2008–2014, the rate in Appalachia was 18 percent higher than the non-Appalachian US rate, signifying a growing disparity.

Indicator 4: Stroke

Between 1989–1995 and 2008–2014, the stroke mortality rate in Appalachia declined by 35 percent, compared with a 41 percent decrease in the non-Appalachian United States. Despite the region's improvement, the gap between Appalachia and the rest of the country increased between the two periods. During 1989–1995, the stroke mortality rate in Appalachia was only 5 percent higher than the rate in the rest of the United States; by 2008–2014, the rate in Appalachia was 15 percent higher than the non-Appalachian US rate, signifying a growing disparity.

Indicator 5: Infant Mortality

Between 1989–1995 and 2008–2014, the infant mortality rate in Appalachia decreased by 19 percent, which was less than the 28 percent decrease in the rest of the country. Despite the region's improvement, the gap between Appalachia and the non-Appalachian United States increased between the two

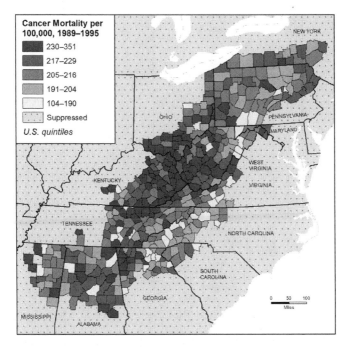

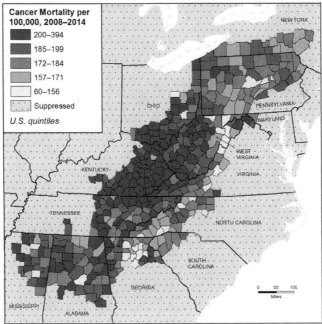

Figure 3.2. Cancer mortality rates in the Appalachian region, 1989–1995 and 2008–2014. (*Source:* Julie L. Marshall et al., *Health Disparities in Appalachia* [Washington, DC: ARC, 2017])

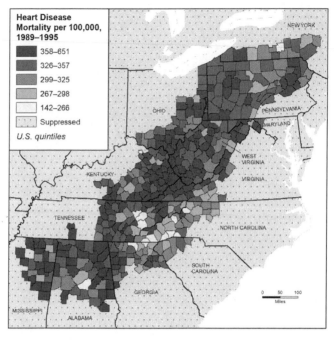

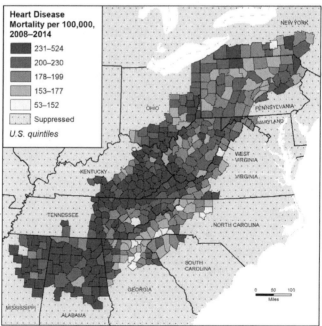

Figure 3.3. Heart disease mortality rates in the Appalachian region, 1989–1995 and 2008–2014. (*Source:* Julie L. Marshall et al., *Health Disparities in Appalachia* [Washington, DC: ARC, 2017])

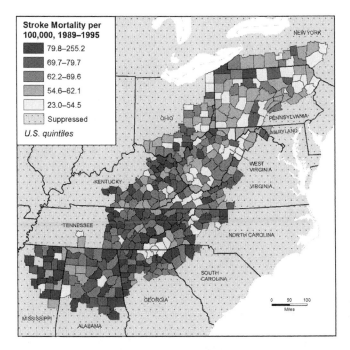

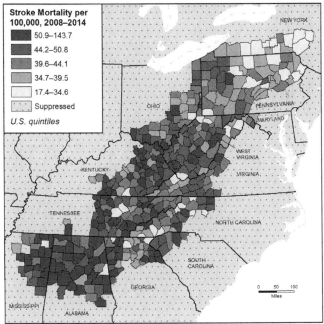

Figure 3.4. Stroke mortality rates in the Appalachian region, 1989–1995 and 2008–2014. (*Source:* Julie L. Marshall et al., *Health Disparities in Appalachia* [Washington, DC: ARC, 2017])

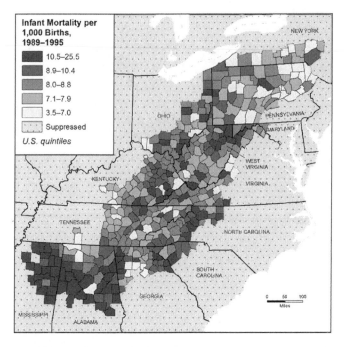

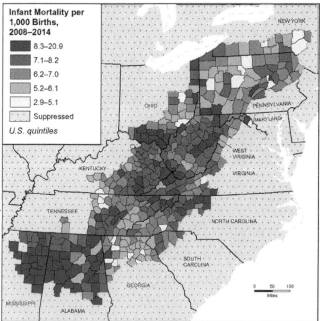

Figure 3.5. Infant mortality rates in the Appalachian region, 1989–1995 and 2008–2014. (*Source:* Julie L. Marshall et al., *Health Disparities in Appalachia* [Washington, DC: ARC, 2017])

periods. During 1989–1995, the infant mortality rate in Appalachia was only 4 percent higher than the rate in the rest of the United States; by 2008–2014, the rate in Appalachia was 16 percent higher than in the rest of the country, signifying a growing disparity.

Of the fifteen indicators featured in this chapter, the Appalachian region performed better than the rest of the United States on just one: HIV prevalence. For each of the remaining fourteen indicators, Appalachia's performance was worse than that of the rest of the country.

For seven of the ten leading causes of death in the United States (heart disease, cancer, injury, COPD, stroke, diabetes, and suicide), Appalachia had higher mortality rates than the rest of the United States. Mortality due to poisoning, which includes drug overdoses, was markedly higher in the region than in the rest of the country. YPLL, a broad measure of premature mortality, was also higher in Appalachia.

Appalachia does not fare much better when it comes to measures of morbidity. The average number of both physically and mentally unhealthy days was higher in Appalachia than elsewhere in the United States. The prevalence of diabetes and adult obesity was also higher.

In terms of changes in five measures—heart disease mortality, cancer mortality, stroke mortality, infant mortality, and YPLL—over the past twenty years, Appalachia experienced improvements in all five measures. However, the region's progress lagged behind that made in the rest of the country, resulting in widening disparities in health outcomes between Appalachia and the non-Appalachian United States.

Notes

This chapter is based on a previously published report: Julie L. Marshall et al., *Health Disparities in Appalachia* (Washington, DC: ARC, 2017).

1. Gopal K. Singh, Michael D. Kogan, and Rebecca T. Slifkin, "Widening Disparities in Infant Mortality and Life Expectancy between Appalachia and the Rest of the United States, 1990–2013," *Health Affairs* 36, no. 8 (2017): 1423–32; Julie L. Marshall et al., *Health Disparities in Appalachia* (Washington, DC: ARC, 2017).

2. Unless otherwise noted, descriptions of the indicators, including definitions and sources, are from Marshall et al., *Health Disparities in Appalachia*.

3. See Marshall et al., *Health Disparities in Appalachia*, 378, for a detailed description of the levels of rurality. Metro counties are counties in large metropolitan areas with more than 1 million residents. Rural counties are nonmetropolitan counties that are not adjacent to a metro area. See Marshall et al., *Health Disparities in Appalachia*, 25, for details on the Appalachian subregions.

4. Melodie Heron, "Deaths: Leading Causes for 2017," *National Vital Statistics Reports* 68, no. 6 (2019): 1–77, https://www.cdc.gov/nchs/data/nvsr/nvsr68/nvsr68_06-508.pdf; Cheryl D. Fryar, Te-Ching Chen, and Xianfen Li, *Prevalence of Uncontrolled Risk Factors for Cardiovascular Disease: United States, 1999–2010,* NCHS Data Brief 103 (Hyattsville, MD: National Center for Health Statistics, Centers for Disease Control and Prevention, US Department of Health and Human Services, 2012).

5. Heron, "Deaths: Leading Causes for 2017," 1; Hanna K. Weir et al., "Heart Disease and Cancer Deaths—Trends and Projections in the United States, 1969–2020," *Preventing Chronic Disease, Public Health Research, Practice, and Policy* 157, no. 157 (2016): 1–10, https://doi.org/10.5888/pcd13.160211; Michael C. Harding et al., "Transitions from Heart Disease to Cancer as the Leading Cause of Death in US States, 1999–2016," *Preventing Chronic Disease* 15, no. 180151 (2018), http://dx.doi.org/10.5888/pcd15.180151; CDC, "How to Prevent Cancer or Find It Early," July 9, 2019, https://www.cdc.gov/cancer/dcpc/prevention/index.htm; US Department of Justice, Drug Enforcement Administration, *2018 National Drug Threat Assessment* (Washington, DC: US Department of Justice, DEA, 2018), v, https://www.dea.gov/sites/default/files/2018-11/DIR-032-18%202018%20NDTA%20final%20low%20resolution.pdf.

6. Michael Meit, Megan Heffernan, and Erin Tanenbaum, "Investigating the Impact of the Diseases of Despair in Appalachia," *Journal of Appalachian Health* 1, no. 2 (2019): 7–18, https://doi.org/10.13023/jah.0102.02; Kate Beatty et al., *Issue Brief: Health Disparities Related to Opioid Misuse in Appalachia: Practical Strategies and Recommendations for Communities* (Washington, DC: ARC, 2019), 3.

7. Heron, "Deaths: Leading Causes for 2017," 1; CDC, "What Is COPD?" June 6, 2018, https://www.cdc.gov/copd/index.html; Linus H. Santo Tomas, "Emphysema and Chronic Obstructive Pulmonary Disease in Coal Miners," *Current Opinion in Pulmonary Medicine* 17, no. 2 (2011): 123–25; A. Scott Laney and David N. Weissman, "Respiratory Diseases Caused by Coal Mine Dust," *Journal of Occupational and Environmental Medicine* 56, suppl. 10 (2014): S18–22; Eileen D. Kuempel et al., "Contributions of Dust Exposure and Cigarette Smoking to Emphysema Severity in Coal Miners in the United States," *American Journal of Respiratory and Critical Care Medicine* 180, no. 3 (2009): 257–64.

8. Heron, "Deaths: Leading Causes for 2017," 1; Amelia K. Boehme, Charles Esenwa, and Mitchell S. V. Elkind, "Stroke Factors, Genetics, and Prevention," *Circulation Research* 120, no. 3 (2017): 472–95; Jonathan Emberson et al., "Effect of Treatment Delay, Age, and Stroke Severity on the Effects of Intravenous Thrombolysis with Alteplase for Acute Ischaemic Stroke: A Meta-analysis of Individual Patient Data from Randomized Trials," *Lancet* 384, no. 9958 (2014): 1929–35; Quanhe Yang Xin Tong et al., "Vital Signs: Recent Trends in Stroke Death Rates—United States, 2000–2015," *Morbidity and Mortality Weekly Report* 66, no. 35 (2017): 933–39.

9. Heron, "Deaths: Leading Causes for 2017," 1; Laura N. McEwen et al., "Diabetes Reporting as a Cause of Death," *Diabetes Care* 29, no. 2 (2006): 247–53; Jose Miguel Baena-Diez et al., "Risk of Cause-Specific Death in Individuals with Diabetes: A Competing Risks Analysis," *Diabetes Care* 39, no. 11 (2016): 1987–95; CDC, "Prevent Complications," August 1, 2019, https://www.cdc.gov/diabetes/managing/problems.html.

10. Heron, "Deaths: Leading Causes for 2017," 1; CDC, "Risk and Protective Factors," September 3, 2019, https://www.cdc.gov/violenceprevention/suicide/riskprotectivefactors.html; Elizabeth Maloney et al., "Suicidal Behaviour and Associated Risk Factors among Opioid-Dependent Individuals: A Case-Control Study," *Addiction* 102, no. 12 (2007): 1933–41.

11. Holly Hedegaard, Sally C. Curtin, and Margaret Warner, "Suicide Rates in the United States Continue to Increase," *NCHS Data Brief* 309 (2018): 1–8, https://www.cdc .gov/nchs/data/databriefs/db309.pdf; Anne Case and Angus Deaton, "Rising Morbidity and Mortality in Midlife among White Non-Hispanic Americans in the 21st Century," *Proceedings of the National Academy of Sciences of the United States of America* 112, no. 49 (2015): 15078–83; National Institute of Mental Health, "Suicide," April 2019, https://www .nimh.nih.gov/health/statistics/suicide.shtml#part_154971; Cynthia A. Fontanella et al., "Widening Rural-Urban Disparities in Youth Suicides, United States, 2016," *JAMA Pediatrics* 169, no. 5 (2015): 466–73.

12. D. D. Reidpath and P. Allotey, "Infant Mortality Rate as an Indicator of Population Health," *Journal of Epidemiology and Community Health* 57, no. 5 (2003): 344–46; CDC, "Infant Mortality," March 27, 2019, https://www.cdc.gov/reproductivehealth/maternalinfanthealth/infantmortality.htm; CDC, "Maternal and Infant Health," September 3, 2019, https://www.cdc.gov/reproductivehealth/maternalinfanthealth/index.html.

13. County Health Rankings & Roadmaps, "Premature Death (YPLL)," RWJF, 2020, https://www.countyhealthrankings.org/explore-health-rankings/measures-data-sources /county-health-rankings-model/health-outcomes/length-of-life/premature-death-ypll; Elizabeth Dranger and Patrick Remington, "YPLL: A Summary Measure of Premature Mortality Used in Measuring the Health of Communities," *Wisconsin Public Health and Health Policy Institute Issue Brief* 5, no. 7 (2004): 1–2.

14. See Marshall et al., *Health Disparities in Appalachia,* for the underlying rural and metro data for each indicator.

15. See Marshall et al., *Health Disparities in Appalachia,* for the underlying subregion data for each indicator.

16. CDC, *Measuring Healthy Days* (Atlanta: CDC, 2000); Anastasia F. Hutchinson et al., "Relationship between Health-Related Quality of Life, Comorbidities and Acute Health Care Utilization, in Adults with Chronic Conditions," *Health and Quality of Life Outcomes* 13, no. 69 (2015): 1–10; H. Jia, P. Muenning, E. I. Lubetkin, and M. R. Gold, "Predicting Geographical Variations in Behavioural Risk Factors: An Analysis of Physical and Mental Health Days," *Journal of Epidemiology and Community Health* 58 (2004): 150–55.

17. Jia et al., "Predicting Geographical Variations," 154; America's Health Rankings, "Poor Mental Health Days," United Health Foundation, 2019, https://www.americashealthrankings .org/explore/senior/measure/mental_health_days_sr/population/mental_health_days _sr_HS_Grad/state/ALL; National Institute of Mental Health, "Chronic Illness and Mental Health," 2019, https://www.nimh.nih.gov/health/publications/chronic-illness-mental-health /index.shtml.

18. CDC, "Basic Statistics," August 6, 2019, https://www.cdc.gov/hiv/basics/statistics .html; CDC, "HIV Transmission," August 6, 2019, https://www.cdc.gov/hiv/basics/transmission.html; CDC, "HIV and Viral Hepatitis," June 2017, https://www.cdc.gov/hiv/pdf /library/factsheets/hiv-viral-hepatitis.pdf; CDC, "TB and HIV Coinfection," March 15, 2016, https://www.cdc.gov/tb/topic/basics/tbhivcoinfection.htm; Michelle M. Van Handel et al., "County-Level Vulnerability Assessment for Rapid Dissemination of HIV or HCV Infections among Persons Who Inject Drugs, United States," *Journal of Acquired Immune Deficiency Syndromes* 73, no. 3 (2016): 323–31.

19. CDC, *National Diabetes Statistics Report, 2020: Estimates of Diabetes and Its Burden in the United States* (Washington, DC: CDC, 2020), https://www.cdc.gov/diabetes/pdfs /data/statistics/national-diabetes-statistics-report.pdf; CDC, "About Prediabetes and Type

2 Diabetes," April 4, 2019, https://www.cdc.gov/diabetes/prevention/lifestyle-program /about-prediabetes.html; CDC, "Putting the Brakes on Diabetes Complications," December 21, 2017, https://www.cdc.gov/features/preventing-diabetes-complications/index.html; CDC, "Prevent Complications"; Shilpa N. Bhupathiraju and Frank B. Hu, "Epidemiology of Obesity and Diabetes and Their Cardiovascular Complications," *Circulation Research* 118, no. 111 (2016): 1723–35; A. O'Connor and G. Wellenius, "Rural-Urban Disparities in the Prevalence of Diabetes and Coronary Heart Disease," *Public Health* 126, no. 10 (2012): 813–20; CDC, "Who's at Risk?" August 28, 2019, https://www.cdc.gov/diabetes/basics /risk-factors.html.

20. CDC, "Behavior, Environment, and Genetic Factors All Have a Role in Causing People to Be Overweight," January 19, 2018, https://www.cdc.gov/genomics/resources /diseases/obesity/index.htm; CDC, "Adult Obesity Causes and Consequences," August 29, 2017, https://www.cdc.gov/obesity/adult/causes.html; CDC, "Adult Obesity Facts," August 13, 2018, https://www.cdc.gov/obesity/data/adult.html; Cynthia L. Ogden, Margaret D. Carroll, Cheryl D. Fryar, and Katherine M. Glegal, *Prevalence of Obesity among Adults and Youth: United States, 2011–2014*, NCHS Data Brief 2019 (Hyattsville, MD: National Center for Health Statistics, 2015), 1–8, https://www.cdc.gov/nchs/data/databriefs/db219.pdf.

21. See Marshall et al., *Health Disparities in Appalachia,* for the subregion data for each indicator.

22. See Marshall et al., *Health Disparities in Appalachia,* for the underlying rural and metro data for each indicator.

23. Marshall et al., *Health Disparities in Appalachia,* 319–34.

4

The Social Determinants of Health

Kate Beatty and Melissa White

The social determinants of health (SDOH) are defined by the Centers for Disease Control and Prevention (CDC) as the "conditions in the places where people live, learn, work, and play [that] affect a wide range of health risks and outcomes." The SDOH may be defined either by place (e.g., school, work, neighborhood, faith community) or by the degree of social interaction people have within each place. This chapter describes the SDOH and how they affect the lives of people living in Appalachia. It also provides examples of grassroots efforts across the Appalachian region to address the SDOH.[1]

Definition of SDOH

Healthy People 2020 divides the SDOH into five overarching and interconnected determinants: economic stability, education, health and health care, neighborhood and the built environment, and the social and community context in which people live. Economic stability encompasses such factors as poverty, employment, food security, and housing stability. Education includes early education and development, high school graduation, enrollment in higher education, and language and literacy. Health and health care primarily reflect access to health care, including primary care and mental health providers; access to and utilization of insurance; and health literacy. Neighborhood and the built environment include the physical conditions in which people live, crime and violence, quality of housing, and access to food that supports healthy eating patterns. Finally, the social and community context includes issues associated with social cohesion and civic participation, as well as discrimination and incarceration rates.[2]

Understanding of the impact of SDOH on health outcomes has increased significantly over the past thirty years. The Whitehall study in the 1980s identified a significant mortality gradient between different grades (i.e., levels) of British civil servants. Subsequent work by Marmot and others has documented variations in health across social conditions in other settings.[3] In their seminal article "The Actual Causes of Death in the United States," McGinnis and Foege reported that social circumstances account for about 15 percent of premature deaths in the country.[4]

Subsequent reports documented that many unhealthy behaviors are dis-proportionately represented in lower socioeconomic groups in the United States, making it clear that health behaviors do not occur in isolation but are impacted by the social context. Behaviors such as smoking, lack of physical activity, and use of illegal substances are all more common in poorer commu-nities.[5] It has also been documented that lower educational achievement, adverse childhood experiences, lack of access to healthy food, and lack of access to primary care are all more common in poorer communities.[6] The effects of socioeconomic status on health are well known and have been thor-oughly documented. Simply put, greater wealth is associated with better health outcomes in most areas, both domestically and internationally. These interre-lationships make it extremely important to consider the full range of medical, behavioral, and social factors that affect a community to both understand the health challenges of that community and construct a rational approach to moving forward.[7]

Methods

To assess the SDOH in Appalachia, data were gathered from various sources, including the American Community Survey, County Health Rankings, Annual Survey of Jails, Institute of Health Metrics and Evaluation, and Appalachian Regional Commission's (ARC's) economic status designations. The county-level data included 2,714 non-Appalachian counties, 420 Appalachian coun-ties, and 8 stand-alone cities in Virginia. Appalachian counties and cities were divided into subregions to assess variability in health outcomes, health behav-iors, poverty, educational achievement, social isolation and cohesion, the built environment, and health insurance and health care within the region. When comparing the non-Appalachian United States to Appalachia as a whole, t-tests were used to compare the means of these two groups for each variable assessed. Analysis of variance (ANOVA) tests were used to compare the means of the subregions within Appalachia to each other as well as to the non-Appalachian United States. Additionally, ARC economic status designations were utilized to separate Appalachian counties based on economic stability. ANOVA tests were used to compare the variability of the means of the aforementioned indicators based on these economic status groups within Appalachia alone.[8]

Educational Achievement

Researchers suggest that education is "the principal pathway to financial secu-rity, stable employment, and social success." Access to education and the qual-ity of education vary, depending on the social conditions in which people live,

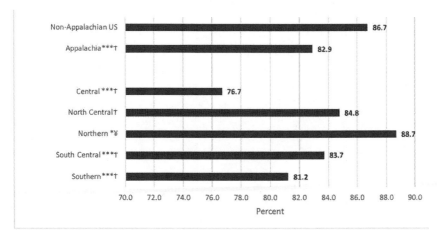

Figure 4.1. Percentage of population with a high school diploma or equivalent, Appalachia versus non-Appalachian United States.

Data from the American Community Survey (2013–2017 five-year estimates).

*, $p < 0.05$; **, $p < 0.01$; ***, $p < 0.001$; ¥, "better" than the non-Appalachian United States; ₮, "worse" than the non-Appalachian United States.

including their neighborhood environment and socioeconomic status. This variation in educational opportunity, in concert with education's role in social success, contributes to an unequal distribution of health. Substantial disparities in educational attainment exist between Appalachia, where 82.9 percent of adults have earned high school diplomas, and the rest of the United States, where 86.7 percent are high school graduates ($p < 0.001$).[9] There are also disparities across the five subregions of Appalachia (see the map of subregions in the front matter). The Northern subregion has the highest percentage of adults with high school diplomas (88.7 percent), slightly higher than the percentage in the non-Appalachian United States ($p < 0.05$), while the Central subregion has the lowest percentage (76.7 percent; $p < 0.001$) (figure 4.1).[10]

Case Study 4.1: The Niswonger Foundation
Nancy Dishner

A desire to have a positive impact on rural Appalachia must include a focus on education. This can be particularly challenging given that, both historically and traditionally, families have often downplayed the importance of educational attainment. Some families may see education as a potentially divisive factor in maintaining the established culture of their family units. Other parents may want their children to have the opportunities offered by more education but lack the skill and confidence to help them navigate a postsecondary experience.

Beyond these cultural concerns, rural communities must often struggle with resource constraints that limit the ability to provide quality educational opportunities. For example, it is more challenging to recruit teachers and school leaders to rural areas when urban areas offer higher salaries and a better perceived lifestyle. This is particularly true for disciplines such as science, math, international languages, and special education.

The Niswonger Foundation, a private educational foundation established in 2001 by businessman and philanthropist Scott M. Niswonger, has a well-established history of supporting solutions that improve educational attainment in even the most rural settings. The foundation's philosophy is that progress in improving educational experiences in rural schools must focus on rigorous classroom instruction, professional learning opportunities for educators (teachers, paraprofessionals, and school leadership), research-based activities, cost-effective project designs, sustainable programs, and, importantly, working in partnership. Examples follow:

- Collaboration leverages the strength of rural communities. The Niswonger Consortium comprises seventeen school systems spanning the First Congressional District of northeastern Tennessee. The foundation sees its primary responsibility as uniting the leadership of these systems in mutually beneficial collaboration. For instance, leadership meetings focus on priorities that can benefit all or most of the school systems. For some projects, the school systems join the Niswonger Foundation in providing financial support. In addition to the foundation's endowment, private, state, and federal grants are sought, leveraging the strength of the regional partnership.
- Professional learning opportunities are shared across the consortium. Professional learning days bring educators from across the region together to learn best practices and be inspired by nationally recognized keynote speakers. Regional training focuses on areas of need, including support for new school leaders and effective use of classroom technology. The Advanced Placement (AP)

Program unites the region's teachers with their subject-area colleagues.

- A focus on rigorous and effective classroom instruction includes projects to improve literacy in the early and middle grades. The Niswonger Consortium also has a well-established online high school program with more than forty courses taught by the region's best educators. These courses span the curriculum, with special attention given to areas in which finances and teacher availability may limit access (e.g., AP and international languages). The Niswonger Foundation has supported more than 500 teachers' AP training.
- Support for underserved students is critical to encouraging rural students to stay in school and graduate. As an example, the Niswonger Foundation has a cadre of college and career advisers that serve the region's thirty high schools, helping students navigate the path to postsecondary education and careers.
- Leadership capacity is fundamental to the foundation's efforts. The Niswonger Scholars Program provides a full scholarship, expansive leadership training, and support for individual development in exchange for a commitment to return to northeastern Tennessee, ensuring leaders for the future.

Dr. Nancy Dishner is president and CEO of the Niswonger Foundation. Visit the website at www.niswongerfoundation.org.

Social Isolation and Cohesion

The cultivation and maintenance of social relationships are imperative for both physical and mental health. The lack of social relationships (social isolation) is associated with higher all-cause mortality as well as increased rates of negative health behaviors and poor health outcomes. Social cohesion, defined as "the extent of connectedness and solidarity among groups," reflects the strength of these social relationships within a community. Social capital, defined as tangible and intangible resources shared by a group, is a measure of social cohesion. The number of membership or social associations within a community is an estimation of the social capital available to its members (figure 4.2).[11]

An examination of these associations reveals that Appalachia has fewer membership or social associations per 10,000 population compared with the

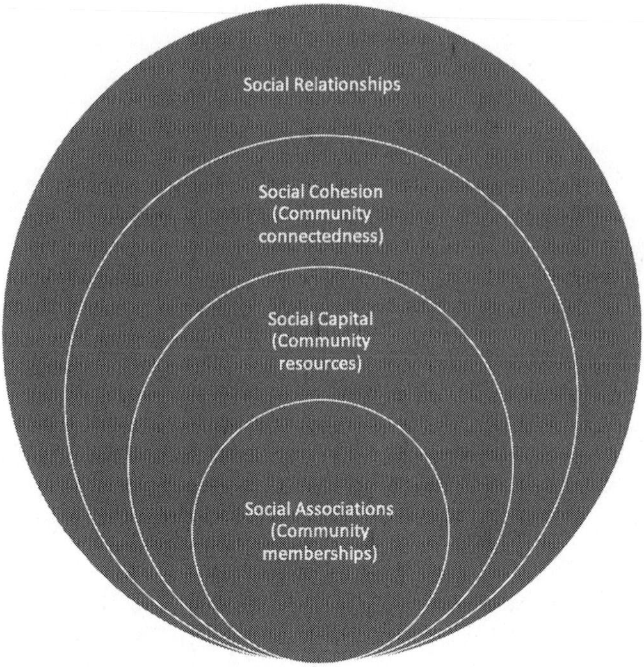

Figure 4.2. Social relationships, social cohesion, social capital, and social associations.

rest of the United States (12.3 and 14.0, respectively; $p < 0.001$) (figure 4.3). Within Appalachia, the Northern subregion has the greatest number of social associations (15.7; $p = 0.241$), exceeding the US average; Central Appalachia has the lowest number of social associations (8.0; $p < 0.001$).

In contrast, a community's incarceration rate—the number of people in local jails, as well as those under the legal authority of state and federal correctional facilities, per 100,000 US population—negatively correlates with social cohesion. A higher incarceration rate is associated with fewer neighborhood social ties or networks. Compared with the rest of the United States, Appalachia's daily average jail count is significantly lower, at 186.7 ($p < 0.001$) (figure 4.4). However, further analysis of the subregions reveals that there is broad variation in the daily average jail count: Southern Appalachia has the highest, at 266.0 (even greater than the US average), and North Central Appalachia has the lowest, with an average daily county jail population of 84.8. These differences may be explained by the region's racial diversity because, unfortunately, black populations are disproportionately incarcerated in the United States. Racial diversity also varies within the region, with Southern

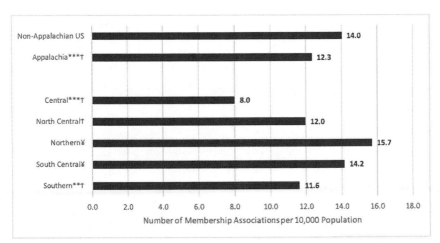

Figure 4.3. Social associations, Appalachia versus non-Appalachian United States.
Data from the County Health Rankings (2019).

$*$, $p < 0.05$; $**$, $p < 0.01$; $***$, $p < 0.001$; ¥, "better" than the non-Appalachian United States; Ŧ, "worse" than the non-Appalachian United States.

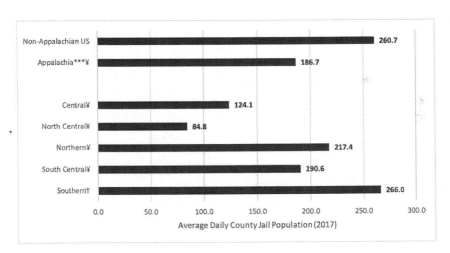

Figure 4.4. Incarceration rate per 100,000 population, Appalachia versus non-Appalachian United States.

Data from the Annual Survey of Jails and Census of Jails (2017), supported by the Vera Institute of Justice Incarceration Trends Dataset and the US Department of Justice's Bureau of Justice Statistics.

$*$, $p < 0.05$; $**$, $p < 0.01$; $***$, $p < 0.001$; ¥, "better" than the non-Appalachian United States; Ŧ, "worse" than the non-Appalachian United States.

Appalachia having the greatest percentage of black non-Hispanic individuals (19.3 percent) and Central Appalachia having the lowest (5.5 percent).[12]

Case Study 4.2. Tennessee Institute of Public Health
Ginny Kidwell

The Tennessee Institute of Public Health (TNIPH) in the East Tennessee State University College of Public Health has a proven track record of facilitating new and existing relationships with community stakeholders. The Correctional Career Pathways (CCP) program in rural Tennessee works with local governments and businesses to lower recidivism among inmates. The first of its kind in the state and possibly in the nation, the CCP program began at the Greene County, Tennessee, Workhouse in April 2015. This program, led by a local multisector leadership team, gives criminal offenders the opportunity to break the cycle of arrest and incarceration and transition into the workforce. It offers classes, job placement, counseling (mental health and substance abuse), transportation, and other services to qualified inmates. After receiving instruction in life skills and special training, trustee inmates go to work at local manufacturing plants or businesses. A certain percentage of the inmate's earnings is set aside to pay court-ordered costs, fines, restitution, and child support. The rest is placed in a savings account for the inmate to use during incarceration and upon release. The TNIPH awards grants to qualified organizations (e.g., sheriff's offices, nonprofits) in local communities to replicate the CCP model and leads a launch team to provide mentorship, oversight, training, and technical assistance in support of these projects. These grants are awarded through a regionwide competitive process.

Ginny Kindwell, MALS, is executive director of TNIPH. Visit the website at https://www.etsu.edu/tniph/default.php.

The Built Environment

The built environment is the physical setting in which people live, including "homes, buildings, streets, open spaces, and infrastructure." It also includes environmental components such as parks, sidewalks, grocery stores, and elements that support or discourage health-promoting or health-limiting behaviors (e.g., access to fresh fruits and vegetables, opportunities for physical activity). Additional information on the built environment is provided in

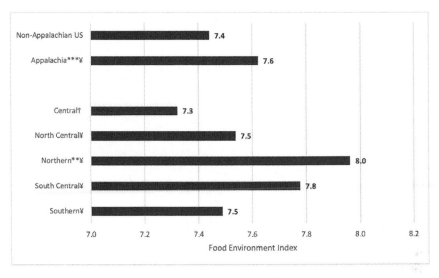

Figure 4.5. Food environment index, Appalachia versus non-Appalachian United States.

Data from the American Community Survey (2013–2017 five-year estimates).

*, $p < 0.05$; **, $p < 0.01$; ***, $p < 0.001$; ¥, "better" than the non-Appalachian United States; ┼, "worse" than the non-Appalachian United States.

chapter 7. The food environment index, which is based on "both proximity to healthy foods and income," provides data on access to healthy food. The Appalachian region has a higher (better) food environment index compared with the rest of the United States, with an overall index score of 7.6 ($p < 0.001$) (figure 4.5). However, consistent with previously mentioned variables, there are great differences in the food environment index among the Appalachian subregions, ranging from a score of 8.0 ($p = 0.001$) in Northern Appalachia to 7.3 ($p = 0.944$) in Central Appalachia.[13]

Case Study 4.3. Appalachian Sustainable Development
Kathlyn Terry Baker

Appalachian Sustainable Development (ASD) is a Central Appalachia–based 501(c)(3) nonprofit that builds entrepreneurial opportunities in the agricultural sector; increases access to fresh, healthy food; and paves the way for people to compete in exciting new market opportunities to generate wealth that remains in the region.

In recognition of the fact that access to healthy food requires gainful employment, ASD focuses much of its work on enhancing the food system to provide economic opportunities for farmers and would-be farmers. This means building scale-appropriate markets and providing farmers with training and assistance to access them. ASD also owns a small fleet of trucks to transport produce from remote areas of Central Appalachia to grocery store distribution centers in the mid-Atlantic. It has a network of partners that enables it to reach farmers in the most remote areas of Central Appalachia, allowing even small-scale farmers to access markets outside the region that pay a premium for locally sourced produce.

Core to ASD's economic development strategies is a recognition that rural communities must be creative about how they do business. Whereas more populated areas have access to diversified markets and abundant populations, rural communities must find innovative ways to work together to ensure that people are fed and farmers can access markets. For example, ASD contracted with a Kentucky food bank to serve as a drop-off site for farmers. The food bank is paid a modest fee, farmers are able to bring their produce to a central location close to their farms, and ASD is able to pick up all the produce at one place. As a bonus, farmers can deliver seconds (produce that does not meet the strict standards of large wholesale buyers) to the food bank at the same time they deliver their high-quality produce. This example highlights how strategies that are mutually beneficial and cost-effective can be more sustainable—a concept that ASD believes is critical for building healthy rural communities.

In addition to building economic opportunities, ASD seeks to reduce food insecurity. Because most farmers in Central Appalachia are small scale and have limited resources, it is not reasonable to ask these farmers to donate food to those in need. Therefore, ASD's food security programs focus on two strategies: (1) reducing both food waste and costs by using seconds to increase farmer income while providing those in need with low-price (but still high-quality) produce; and (2) building self-reliance by teaching people how to grow their own food and ultimately helping larger gardeners access markets that are appropriate to their scale. These strategies not only increase access to and consumption of healthy food but also build social capital and promote "agripreneurism" in rural communities.

Kathlyn Terry Baker is executive director of ASD. Visit the website at https://asdevelop.org/.

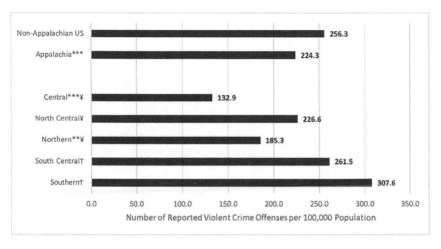

Figure 4.6. Violent crime rate per 100,000 population, Appalachia versus non-Appalachian United States.

Data from the County Health Rankings (2019).

*, $p < 0.05$; **, $p < 0.01$; ***, $p < 0.001$; ¥, "better" than the non-Appalachian United States; Ť, "worse" than the non-Appalachian United States.

Another aspect of the built environment is personal safety, including exposure to violent crime. According to the FBI, violent crime includes "murder and nonnegligent manslaughter, forcible rape, robbery, and aggravated assault." Interestingly, the violent crime rate is lower in Appalachia than in the rest of the United States (224.3 reported violent crime offenses per 100,000 population; $p < 0.001$) (figure 4.6). However, as with other variables, there is great variation in the violent crime rate among the subregions of Appalachia. Southern Appalachia has the highest rate, at 307.6 per 100,000 population ($p = 0.135$), while Central Appalachia has the lowest, at 132.9 ($p < 0.001$).[14]

Health Insurance and Availability of Health Care

Access to health care is part of the Healthy People 2020 initiative and includes "insurance coverage, health services, and timeliness of care." An important facet of access to health care is the availability and accessibility of providers. An adequate number of primary care physicians is associated with reduced rates of low-birth-weight infants, lower overall health care costs, and fewer health disparities within a population. A higher population–to–health care provider ratio is associated with higher rates of adverse health outcomes. In the Appalachian region as a whole, the ratio is 2,895:1 ($p = 0.053$), which is higher than the ratio

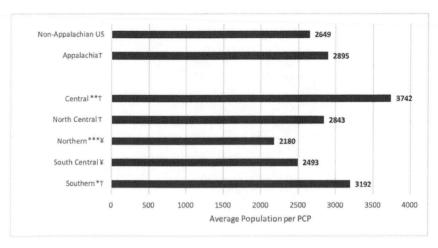

Figure 4.7. Ratio of population to primary care physicians (PCPs), Appalachia versus non-Appalachian United States.

Data from the County Health Rankings (2019).

*, $p < 0.05$; **, $p < 0.01$; ***, $p < 0.001$; ¥, "better" than the non-Appalachian United States; Ϯ, "worse" than the non-Appalachian United States.

in the rest of the United States (figure 4.7). Like other variables, access to primary care providers differs markedly within Appalachia. Northern Appalachia has the lowest average population–to–primary care physician ratio (2,180:1; $p < 0.001$), while Central Appalachia has the highest (3,742:1; $p < 0.01$).[15]

There is great variation in the number of mental health care providers (e.g., psychiatrists and psychologists) between metropolitan and nonmetropolitan areas in the United States. In Appalachia, similar to primary care physicians, the ratio of population to mental health care provider is higher (2,468:1; $p < 0.001$) than in the rest of the United States (1,793:1, $p = 0.005$) (figure 4.8). Southern Appalachia has the highest ratio (3,724:1; $p < 0.001$), while Northern Appalachia has the lowest (1,440:1; $p = 0.797$).[16] See chapter 6 for more information about the availability of health care in Appalachia.

Poverty and Wealth

Poverty has a significant impact on overall health outcomes. As shown in figures 4.9 and 4.10, wealth and poverty vary widely within Appalachia as well as between Appalachia and the rest of the United States. Northern Appalachia has the highest median household income ($49,089.90; $p = 0.798$), while Central Appalachia has the lowest ($34,482.73; $p < 0.001$). Overall, Appalachia has

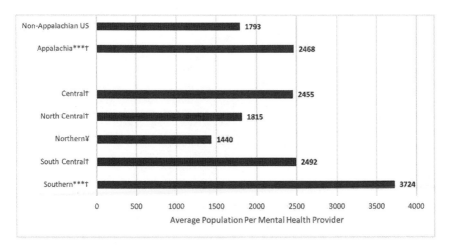

Figure 4.8. Ratio of population to mental health care providers, Appalachia versus non-Appalachian United States.

Data from the County Health Rankings (2019).

*, $p < 0.05$; **, $p < 0.01$; ***, $p < 0.001$; ¥, "better" than the non-Appalachian United States; ₸, "worse" than the non-Appalachian United States.

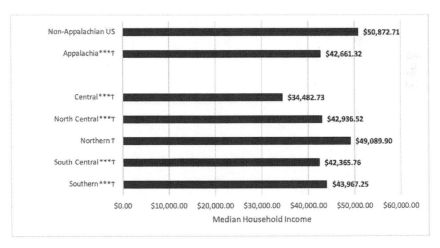

Figure 4.9. Median household income, Appalachia versus non-Appalachian United States.

Data from the American Community Survey (2013–2017 five-year estimates).

*, $p < 0.05$; **, $p < 0.01$; ***, $p < 0.001$; ¥, "better" than the non-Appalachian United States; ₸, "worse" than the non-Appalachian United States.

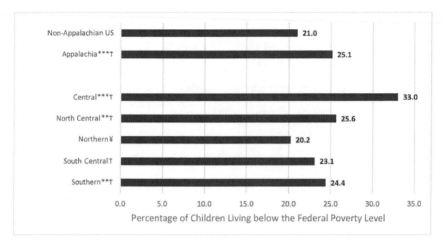

Figure 4.10. Percentage of children living in poverty, Appalachia versus non-Appalachian United States.

Data from the County Health Rankings (2019).

*, $p < 0.05$; **, $p < 0.01$; ***, $p < 0.001$; ¥, "better" than the non-Appalachian United States; ᵀ, "worse" than the non-Appalachian United States.

a lower median household income ($42,661.32; $p < 0.001$) than the rest of the United States.[17]

Childhood poverty has both short- and long-term health consequences, including reduced physical and mental well-being, lower educational achievement, and decreased career success. Poverty inhibits parents and caregivers from accessing certain resources and therefore reduces their ability to share those resources with children. Childhood poverty is also associated with familial and childhood stress, which is related to adverse health outcomes and may affect physiological, psychological, and mental development. Northern Appalachia has the lowest percentage of children living below the federal poverty level (20.2 percent;, $p = 0.968$), and Central Appalachia has the highest percentage (33.0 percent; $p < 0.001$), compared with 21.0 percent in the non-Appalachian United States ($p < 0.001$) (figure 4.10).[18]

Moving from Geography to Economic Indicators

Recent studies have found great variations in economic status within the states, and this is also true within Appalachia. To assess economic stability and overall socioeconomic status, the ARC developed an index that incorporates county-level per capita market income, poverty rate, and unemployment rate in one indicator. Counties are ranked from 1 (best) to 3,113 (worst) and then placed on an economic status spectrum with the following designations: distressed (lowest-ranking 10 percent of counties), at risk (between the lowest 10 percent and 25 percent), transitional (between the lowest 25 percent and highest 25 percent), competitive (between the highest 25 percent and 10 percent), and attainment (highest-ranking 10 percent of counties).[19]

Shaw and colleagues assessed the relationship between socioeconomic status and chronic disease outcomes, while controlling for metropolitan designation (i.e., metro versus nonmetro). Counties with lower socioeconomic status had higher rates of adverse health outcomes, regardless of metropolitan designation. Examining counties in this way helps delineate the relationship between geography and health outcomes and can highlight the impact of economic stability on health. As shown in table 4.1, distressed counties generally have greater rates of adverse health outcomes, worse health-related behaviors, greater poverty, lower educational achievement, fewer beneficial built environment factors, and lower rates of health insurance coverage and health care provider access. Interestingly, distressed counties are concentrated in the Central Appalachian subregion, supporting the data presented in table 4.2, which suggest that these measures are generally worse in the Central subregion.[20]

Table 4.1. Social Determinants of Health, Health Behaviors, and Health Outcomes: ARC Economic Status Designations

	Distressed Appalachia (n=81)	At-Risk Appalachia (n=111)	Transitional Appalachia (n=223)	Competitive + Attainment Appalachia (n=13)
	Mean	Mean	Mean	Mean
Health Outcomes				
Female life expectancy[a,e]	77.1	78.3	79.7	80.8
Male life expectancy[a,e]	71.4	72.8	74.9	76.6
Years of potential life lost[a]	12251	10556	8822	6929
Drug overdose mortality rate[a]	37.5	29.0	26.2	30.7
Diabetes[c]	15.0	14.6	12.8	11.1
Cardiovascular disease mortality[e]	355.4	325.9	288.3	257.5
Cancer mortality[e]	264.7	234.0	215.0	191.4
Health Behaviors				
Adult smoking[c]	24.3	21.2	18.9	16.3
Adult obesity[c]	36.7	34.9	32.7	30.3
Physical inactivity[c]	32.0	30.5	26.6	23.2

	Distressed Appalachia (n=81)	At-Risk Appalachia (n=111)	Transitional Appalachia (n=223)	Competitive + Attainment Appalachia (n=13)
	Mean	Mean	Mean	Mean
Poverty and Wealth				
Median household income ($)[b]	33,168	39,018	46,665	64,246
Population below poverty level[b]	26.4	20.4	15.8	9.5
Children in poverty[a,c]	35.4	27.3	21.1	12.1
Educational Achievement				
High school graduate or higher[b]	76.5	81.3	85.8	88.0
Bachelor's degree or higher[b]	12.2	14.8	20.2	29.7
Social Isolation and Cohesion				
Social associations[c]	8.4	12.2	13.8	13.6
Incarceration rate[a,d]	97.8	110.0	242.2	400.7
Disconnected youth[a,c]	14.2	12.3	8.3	6.1
Black/white residential segregation[a,c]	51.7	44.6	49.3	41.8
Nonwhite/white residential segregation[a,c]	38.0	32.3	34.7	34.7
Built Environment				
Food environment index[a,c]	7.0	7.5	7.9	8.4
Access to exercise opportunities[a,c]	51.6	54.0	66.9	75.2
Severe housing problems[c]	13.9	13.7	13.5	11.8
Air pollution[a,c]	9.8	10.0	10.0	10.7
Violent crime[a,c]	165.6	216.7	252.4	153.8
Limited access to healthy foods[a,c]	5.4	5.2	6.1	7.0
Homicide rate[a,c]	10.0	6.8	4.7	2.9
Firearm fatality rate[a,c]	20.8	17.9	14.6	11.0
Health Insurance/Health Care				
Population–to–primary care physician ratio[a,c]	4161	3341	2289	1948
Population–to–mental health provider ratio[a,c]	2250	3328	2127	2155
Population-to-dentist ratio[a,c]	4841	4222	3151	2354
Adult uninsured rate[a,c]	10.8	13.6	12.1	10.7
Child uninsured rate[a,c]	3.8	4.5	4.5	5.8

[a]N < displayed number
[b]US Census Bureau: American Community Survey (five-year estimates), 2013–2017
[c]County Health Rankings, 2019
[d]Bureau of Justice Statistics, 2017
[e]Institute of Health Metrics and Evaluation, 2014

Table 4.2. Social Determinants of Health, Health Behaviors, and Health Outcomes: Non-Appalachian United States versus Appalachia

	Non-Appalachian US (n=2714)	Appalachia (n=428)	Central Appalachia (n=83)	Northern Appalachia (n=86)	North Central Appalachia (n=63)	Southern Appalachia (n=104)	South Central Appalachia (n=92)
	Mean	Mean	Mean	Mean	Mean	Mean	Mean
Health Outcomes							
Female life expectancy[a,e]	80.4	78.9	77.1	80.8	78.9	78.4	79.2
Male life expectancy[a,e]	75.6	73.7	71.4	76.2	74.1	73.0	75.6
Years of potential life lost[a]	8291	9875	12165	7946	9793	9918	9610
Drug overdose mortality rate[a]	19.9	28.8	36.7	29.0	39.1	17.8	25.3
Diabetes[c]	11.3	13.6	14.9	12.0	14.3	14.2	12.9
Cardiovascular disease mortality[e]	272.8	309.8	356.3	279.8	299.7	318.8	292.6
Cancer mortality[e]	202.9	228.6	267.2	206.3	229.2	227.3	215.6
Health Behaviors							
Adult smoking[c]	17.5	20.4	24.1	17.8	22.2	19.3	19.6
Adult obesity[c]	31.8	34.0	36.0	33.0	36.1	34.2	312
Physical inactivity[c]	25.3	28.5	32.2	25.5	28.5	29.5	27.0
Poverty and Wealth							
Median household income ($)[b]	50,873	42,661	34,483	49,090	42,937	43,967	42,366
Population below poverty level[b]	15.5	18.8	25.2	14.2	18.4	18.5	17.8
Children in poverty[a,c]	21.0	25.1	33.0	20.2	25.6	24.4	23.1
Educational Achievement							
High school graduate or higher[b]	86.7	83.0	76.7	88.7	84.8	81.2	83.7
Bachelor's degree or higher[b]	21.8	17.6	12.4	20.3	16.3	18.5	19.4
Social Isolation and Cohesion							
Social associations[c]	14.0	12.3	8.0	15.7	12.0	11.6	14.2
Incarceration rate[a,d]	260.7	186.7	124.1	217.4	84.8	266.0	190.6

	Non-Appalachian US (n=2714)	Appalachia (n=428)	Central Appalachia (n=83)	Northern Appalachia (n=86)	North Central Appalachia (n=63)	Southern Appalachia (n=104)	South Central Appalachia (n=92)
	Mean	Mean	Mean	Mean	Mean	Mean	Mean
Disconnected youth[a,c]	9.3	9.5	12.0	7.5	10.9	10.1	10.2
Black/white residential segregation[a,c]	45.0	48.1	57.9	59.2	48.8	37.5	45.8
Nonwhite/white residential segregation[a,c]	30.4	34.6	37.1	38.6	36.1	31.1	31.8
Built Environment							
Food environment index[a,c]	7.4	7.6	7.3	8.0	7.5	7.5	7.8
Access to exercise opportunities[a,c]	63.2	60.9	53.5	70.2	55.6	54.4	70.0
Severe housing problems[c]	14.3	13.5	14.0	12.9	11.6	14.7	13.8
Air pollution[a,c]	8.9	10.0	9.9	10.2	9.8	10.7	9.4
Violent crime[a,c]	256.3	224.3	132.9	185.3	226.6	307.6	261.5
Limited access to healthy foods[a,c]	9.1	5.8	3.9	5.3	6.7	6.3	6.6
Homicide rate[a,c]	6.5	5.7	6.7	3.7	5.7	7.1	4.9
Firearm fatality rate[a,c]	15.0	16.4	19.9	11.8	16.5	17.6	16.6
Health Insurance/Health Care							
Population–to–primary care physician ratio[a,c]	2649	2895	3742	2180	2843	3192	2493
Population–to–mental health provider ratio[a,c]	1793	2468	2455	1440	1815	3724	2492
Population-to-dentist ratio[a,c]	2948	2716	4647	2726	3314	4412	3304
Adult uninsured rate[a,c]	13.5	12.2	9.9	7.5	8.4	17.7	15.0
Child uninsured rate[a,c]	6.1	4.4	3.8	4.5	3.1	5.3	4.8

[a]N < displayed number

[b]US Census Bureau: American Community Survey (five-year estimates), 2013–2017

[c]County Health Rankings, 2019

[d]Bureau of Justice Statistics, 2017

[e]Institute of Health Metrics and Evaluation, 2014

Ideally, only 10 percent (about 43) of all Appalachian counties and cities (428) should be considered economically distressed. However, as seen in table 4.1, there are 81 distressed counties in Appalachia (19 percent), almost twice the expected number. Further, this unevenness translates into worse health outcomes and behaviors in these economically distressed and at-risk counties. These data provide compelling evidence that the relationship between socioeconomic indicators and adverse health outcomes should be examined not only at the regional and subregional levels but also at the county level.

Using the SDOH to better understand health care in Appalachia exemplifies why the improvement of regional health outcomes is fraught with challenges. As noted in chapter 2, difficult social conditions abound in Appalachia, and a litany of stereotypes tends to color the region monochromatically. Yet this subregional analysis reveals great diversity at the county level. Even social conditions that have become synonymous with Appalachia—such as poverty and low educational attainment—occur unevenly. Central Appalachia's low median household income and high percentage of childhood poverty are not replicated in Northern Appalachia, for example. This variation complicates efforts to address the region's lagging health outcomes because there is no panacea that will help all communities within all subregions simultaneously. However, the uncovering and understanding of Appalachia's complexities highlight clear areas of opportunity: perhaps policy makers should focus first on interventions to aid the most economically distressed counties, or perhaps they will find success by adapting health interventions for subregional implementation, using the social contexts of these places as a guide.

Notes

1. CDC, "Social Determinants of Health (SDOH)," January 29, 2017, https://www.cdc.gov/socialdeterminants/index.htm.

2. Office of Disease Prevention and Health Promotion, "Social Determinants of Health," https://www.healthypeople.gov/2020/topics-objectives/topic/social-determinants-of-health.

3. Michael G. Marmot, Martin J. Shipley, and Geoffrey Rose, "Inequalities in Death—Specific Explanations of a General Pattern?" *Lancet* 323, no. 8384 (1984): 1003–6; Michael G. Marmot, Manolis Kogevinas, and Mary Ann Elston, "Social/Economic Status and Disease," *Annual Review of Public Health* 8, no. 1 (1987): 111–35; Michael G. Marmot, "Social Differentials in Health within and between Populations," *Daedalus* 123, no. 4 (1994): 197–216.

4. J. Michael McGinnis and William H. Foege, "The Actual Causes of Death in the United States," *JAMA* 270, no. 18 (1993): 2207–12.

5. Olivia Egen et al., "Health and Social Conditions of the Poorest versus Wealthiest Counties in the United States," *American Journal of Public Health* 107, no. 1 (2016): 130–35; National Institute on Drug Abuse, "Health Consequences of Drug Misuse," NIH, March 23, 2017, https://www.drugabuse.gov/related-topics/health-consequences-drug-misuse.

6. Egen et al., "Health and Social Conditions"; Neal Halfon et al., "Income Inequality and the Differential Effect of Adverse Childhood Experiences in US Children," *Academic Pediatrics* 17, no. 7S (2017): S70–78; William Pickett, Valerie Michaelson, and Colleen Davison, "Beyond Nutrition: Hunger and Its Impact on the Health of Young Canadians," *International Journal of Public Health* 60, no. 5 (2015): 527–38.

7. Nancy Adler and Judith Stewart, *Reaching for a Healthier Life: Facts on Socioeconomic Status and Health in the U.S.* (San Francisco: John D. and Catherine T. MacArthur Foundation, 2007); Brian Biggs, Lawrence King, Sanjay Basu, and David Stuckler, "Is Wealthier Always Healthier? The Impact of National Income Level, Inequality, and Poverty on Public Health in Latin America," *Social Science & Medicine* 71, no. 2 (2010): 266–73; Michael G. Marmot, "The Influence of Income on Health: Views of an Epidemiologist," *Health Affairs* 21, no. 2 (2002): 31–46; Michael G. Marmot, *Status Syndrome* (London: Bloomsbury, 2004); John W. Frank et al., "Socioeconomic Gradients in Health Status over 29 Years of Follow-up after Midlife: The Alameda County Study," *Social Science & Medicine* 57, no. 12 (2003): 2305–23; Arline T. Geronimus et al., "Excess Mortality among Blacks and Whites in the United States," *New England Journal of Medicine* 335, no. 21 (1996): 1552–58; Arline T. Geronimus, John Bound, and Timothy A. Waidmann, "Poverty, Time, and Place: Variation in Excess Mortality across Selected US Populations, 1980–1990," *Journal of Epidemiology & Community Health* 53, no. 6 (1999): 325–34; Robert A. Hahn et al., "Poverty and Death in the United States," *International Journal of Health Services* 26, no. 4 (1996): 673–90; Stephen L. Isaacs and Steven A. Schroeder, "Class—The Ignored Determinant of the Nation's Health," *New England Journal of Medicine* 351, no. 11 (2004): 1137–42; Gopal K. Singh, "Area Deprivation and Widening Inequalities in US Mortality, 1969–1998," *American Journal of Public Health* 93, no. 7 (2003): 1137–43; Michael G. Marmot, "Social Determinants of Health Inequalities," *Lancet* 365, no. 9464 (2005): 1099–104.

8. US Census Bureau, "American Community Survey," https://www.census.gov /programs-surveys/acs; County Health Rankings & Roadmaps, "Rankings Data & Documentation," RWJF, https://www.countyhealthrankings.org/explore-health-rankings/rankings -data-documentation; Bureau of Justice Statistics, Office of Justice Programs, "Annual Survey of Jails," 2018, https://www.bjs.gov/index.cfm?ty=dcdetail&iid=261; Institute for Health Metrics and Evaluation, "US County Profiles," http://www.healthdata.org/us-county-profiles; ARC, "Source & Methodology: Distressed Designation and County Economic Status Classification System, FY 2007–2009," 2019, https://www.arc.gov/research/SourceandMethodology CountyEconomicStatusFY2007FY2019.asp.

9. The probability (*p*) values throughout this chapter assess the difference between the Southern Appalachia subregion and the rest of the United States.

10. Anna Zajacova and Elizabeth M. Lawrence, "The Relationship between Education and Health: Reducing Disparities through a Contextual Approach," *Annual Review of Public Health* 39, no. 1 (2018): 273–89.

11. CDC, "Social Determinants of Health"; Nicholas Leigh-Hunt et al., "An Overview of Systematic Reviews on the Public Health Consequences of Social Isolation and Loneliness," *Public Health* 152 (2017): 157–71; Anna Rita Manca, "Social Cohesion," in *Encyclopedia of Quality of Life and Well-Being Research* (Dordrecht: Springer Netherlands, 2014), 6026–28; Office of Disease Prevention and Health Promotion, "Social Cohesion," https://www .healthypeople.gov/2020/topics-objectives/topic/social-determinants-health/interventions -resources/social-cohesion.

12. Jeffrey D. Morenoff and David J. Harding, "Incarceration, Prisoner Reentry, and Communities," *Annual Review of Sociology* 40 (2014): 411–29; Dina R. Rose and Todd R. Clear, "Incarceration, Reentry, and Social Capital: Social Networks in the Balance," in *National Policy Conference: From Prison to Home; the Effect of Incarceration and Reentry on Children, Families and Communities* (Washington, DC: US Department of Health and Human Services and Urban Institute, 2001), https://aspe.hhs.gov/basic-report/incarceration-reentry-and-social-capital-social-networks-balance; Bureau of Justice Statistics, "Key Statistic: Incarceration Rate," 2016, https://www.bjs.gov/index.cfm?ty=kfdetail&iid=493; Christopher Wildeman and Emily A. Wang, "Mass Incarceration, Public Health, and Widening Inequality in the USA," *Lancet* 389, no. 10077 (2017): 1464–74; Kelvin Pollard and Linda A. Jacobsen, *The Appalachian Region: A Data Overview from the 2013–2017 American Community Survey* (Washington, DC: Population Reference Bureau and ARC, 2019), https://www.arc.gov/research/researchreportdetails.asp?REPORT_ID=159.

13. CDC, "Social Determinants of Health"; Andrea Nathan et al., "The Role of the Built Environment on Health across the Life Course: A Call for CollaborACTION," *American Journal of Health Promotion* 32, no. 6 (2018): 1460–68; County Health Rankings & Roadmaps, "Food Environment Index," RWJF, 2020, https://www.countyhealthrankings.org/explore-health-rankings/measures-data-sources/county-health-rankings-model/health-factors/health-behaviors/diet-exercise/food-environment-index.

14. County Health Rankings & Roadmaps, "Violent Crime Rate," RWJF, 2020, https://www.countyhealthrankings.org/explore-health-rankings/measures-data-sources/county-health-rankings-model/health-factors/social-and-economic-factors/community-safety/violent-crime-rate; FBI, "Violent Crime," https://www.countyhealthrankings.org/explore-health-rankings/measures-data-sources/county-health-rankings-model/health-factors/social-and-economic-factors/community-safety/violent-crime-rate.

15. Office of Disease Prevention and Health Promotion, "Access to Health Services," https://www.healthypeople.gov/2020/topics-objectives/topic/Access-to-Health-Services; America's Health Rankings, "Primary Care Physicians, 2019 Annual Report," United Health Foundation, September 23, 2019, https://www.americashealthrankings.org/explore/annual/measure/PCP/state/U.S.; Bronwyn E. Fields, Jeri L. Bigbee, and Janice F. Bell, "Associations of Provider-to-Population Ratios and Population Health by County-Level Rurality," *Journal of Rural Health* 32, no. 3 (2016): 235–44.

16. C. Holly, A. Andrilla, et al., "Geographic Variation in the Supply of Selected Behavioral Health Providers," *American Journal of Preventive Medicine* 6, suppl. 3 (2018): S199–207.

17. Office of Disease Prevention and Health Promotion, "Poverty," https://www.healthypeople.gov/2020/topics-objectives/topic/social-determinants-health/interventions-resources/poverty.

18. National Academies of Sciences, Engineering, and Medicine, "Consequences of Child Poverty," in *A Roadmap to Reducing Child Poverty* (Washington, DC: National Academies Press, 2019), 67–96.

19. Egen et al., "Health and Social Conditions"; Kate Beatty et al., "Poverty and Health in Tennessee," *Southern Medical Journal* 113, no. 1 (2020): 1–7; ARC, "Source & Methodology."

20. ARC, "Distressed Counties Program," https://www.arc.gov/program_areas/index.asp?PROGRAM_AREA_ID=15; Kate M. Shaw et al., "Chronic Disease Disparities by County Economic Status and Metropolitan Classification, Behavioral Risk Factor Surveillance System, 2013," *Preventing Chronic Disease* 13, no. 9 (2013): 160088.

5

Health Behaviors in Appalachia

Robin C. Vanderpool, Angela L. Carman,
Lindsay R. Stradtman, and Kelly D. Blake

Through the power of disease surveillance, the public health community has identified the leading causes of death in the United States, including in specific geographic areas such as the thirteen-state region of Appalachia. The Centers for Disease Control and Prevention (CDC) reported that the top ten leading causes of mortality in 2017 were heart disease, cancer, unintentional injuries, chronic lower respiratory disease, stroke, Alzheimer's disease, diabetes, influenza and pneumonia, kidney disease, and suicide. Notably, heart disease and cancer, which are both highly prevalent throughout Appalachia, are responsible for 46 percent of deaths in the United States each year. Case in point: the fifty-four Appalachian counties in eastern Kentucky lead the nation in both cancer incidence and cancer mortality. Much of eastern Kentucky's cancer burden is attributable to preventable and detectable malignancies such as lung, colorectal, cervical, head and neck cancer, and melanoma. Similarly, recent data published by the Appalachian Regional Commission (ARC) suggest that suicide rates among adults aged fifteen to sixty-four are significantly higher in Appalachia than in other US regions. Notably, one-third of the counties in the nation's "diabetes belt" are in Central and Southern Appalachia, and Appalachian communities' mortality rates from chronic obstructive pulmonary disease (COPD) are 31 percent higher than in the rest of the United States. Although surveillance of these clinical outcomes is important in guiding public health efforts to remediate these problems, it is equally valuable to examine— and intervene in—the underlying behavioral and structural determinants of these leading causes of death in Appalachia.[1]

Through the seminal work of McGinnis and Foege and Mokdad and colleagues, specific modifiable health behaviors have been linked to about half of all mortality outcomes in the United States. This information, in turn, guides the public health community in its population- and individual-level primary and secondary disease prevention efforts. Tobacco use (18.1 percent), physical activity and diet (15.2 percent), and alcohol consumption (3.5 percent) are the top three health behaviors impacting the leading causes of mortality; they contribute to nearly two in five deaths in the United States.[2] Microbial agents, toxic agents, motor vehicle crashes, firearms, certain sexual behaviors, and illicit drug use have been identified as other behavioral risk factors significantly impacting mortality in the United States. In addition, health behaviors that are cognitively oriented (such as health care avoidance, failure to seek health information, and sensation-seeking risk taking) can impede good health. Research scholars, health care professionals, and community leaders readily acknowledge the negative impact these collective behaviors have on health outcomes in Appalachia, including elevated rates of chronic disease and "diseases of despair." As surmised by Farley and Cohen in their thought-provoking *Prescription for a Healthy Nation*, "too many of us smoke, drink alcohol, eat high-calorie and high-fat foods, don't get enough exercise, and use cars and guns to kill ourselves and each other. The major reason why we Americans [and Appalachians] die early is that we behave in an unhealthy way."[3]

Whereas other chapters describe and quantify the clinical disease burden in Appalachia, this chapter presents surveillance data from national, state, regional, and local sources on several prominent and modifiable health behaviors contributing to the significant disease burden in the region. Importantly, this chapter is not an exhaustive assessment of all health behaviors observed among all Appalachian residents. It focuses on three factors because of their substantial impact on health outcomes in Appalachia and our expertise in these areas: tobacco use; physical activity, diet, and weight; and health care avoidance. Other significant behaviors that affect the health of Appalachian populations, such as alcohol and substance use, are discussed in other chapters. Complementing other content in this volume, this chapter also provides a brief commentary on why these selected behaviors are more prevalent in Appalachia than in other US communities. It describes credible sources of evidence-based strategies and interventions aimed at increasing primary and secondary prevention efforts and effecting positive behavioral change. Finally, we provide several examples of Appalachia-focused, evidence-based interventions and programs.[4]

We faced several challenges in describing data and evidence from rural and Appalachia-centric health research and programming. For example, health behavior surveillance data describing the entire thirteen-state Appalachian region are scant compared with state- or local-level data. Additionally, although national and state estimates are commonly published by federal health agencies on an annual basis, Appalachia-specific data are not always recent or timely. Finally, as is true for many other rural or underserved populations, it was difficult to identify evidence-based interventions conducted specifically in Appalachia and thus culturally relevant. With these caveats, we report the evidence from data sets and peer-reviewed studies published within the past ten years and provide multiple examples and cases to illustrate the prevalence and context of particular health behaviors in Appalachian states or subregions. We also describe several innovative interventions and strategies used by Appalachian communities to effect positive behavioral changes in tobacco use; physical activity, diet, and weight; and health care avoidance and to improve related health outcomes in Appalachian populations.[5]

Sources of Appalachia-Specific Health Behavior Data

The CDC's Behavioral Risk Factor Surveillance System (BRFSS), an annual telephone survey, is a resource for population-based data on sociodemographics, chronic disease conditions, health-related behaviors, and the use of preventive services among US adults at the national, state, and metropolitan statistical area levels. The BRFSS counterpart for adolescents is the Youth Risk Behavior Surveillance System (YRBSS), which monitors health behaviors among high school students (grades nine through twelve), including unintentional injuries and violence, sexual behaviors, alcohol and drug use, tobacco use, and diet and physical activity. Other relevant CDC population health surveys include the National Health Interview Survey, National Immunization Surveys (Child, Teens, Adults), and National Health and Nutrition Examination Survey. The National Cancer Institute (NCI) routinely conducts the Health Information National Trends Survey (HINTS), which is a nationally representative assessment of adults' health communication practices and health-related behaviors, particularly those related to cancer risk.[6]

The CDC and NCI provide public-use data sets to researchers and practitioners for secondary data analysis, including Appalachian versus non-Appalachian and within-Appalachia comparisons, typically by state, subregion, economic distress category, or rurality. Appalachia as an analytical geographic region is commonly constructed by identifying those counties designated Appalachian within the various data sets. Additional behavioral health data are commonly collected as part of locally conducted research projects, such as the NCI-funded Population Health Assessment in Cancer Center Catchment Areas initiative conducted by researchers in Kentucky, Ohio, Pennsylvania, and Virginia, as well as other federal, state, regional, and local health initiatives. However, localized data are often limited due to small sample sizes, lack of population representativeness, lack of generalizability to the larger Appalachian region, or inability to compare with other Appalachian or non-Appalachian areas. These are important limitations, given the heterogeneity of Appalachia and its 420 counties and 25 million residents.[7]

Prevalence of Health Behaviors in Appalachia

Tobacco Use

Tobacco use encompasses a range of products, including cigarettes, cigars, smokeless tobacco, hookahs, and electronic cigarettes (e-cigarettes); it is a pervasive health behavior among Appalachian adults and youths. Tobacco use puts individuals and their family members at risk for cancer, respiratory conditions, pregnancy complications, cardiovascular disease, and poor oral health, among other illnesses. Nationally, the goal of Healthy People 2020 was a 12 percent cigarette smoking prevalence rate among adults. However, data from the 2014 BRFSS indicate that 19.8 percent of Appalachian adults (nearly one in five) smoke cigarettes, compared with 16.0 percent of non-Appalachians and 16.3 percent in the United States as a whole. Within Appalachia, the 2014 BRFSS data suggest higher smoking rates among Central (25.2 percent) and North Central (22.8 percent) Appalachian individuals, in rural-designated communities (22.5 percent) versus large metropolitan areas (17.3 percent), and in economically distressed counties (24.7 percent) versus nondistressed counties (19.4 percent). In 2018, West Virginia, which is wholly Appalachian, had the highest rate of adult smokers at 25.3 percent (compared with a median of 16.1 percent nationally). Even higher rates were observed in 2017 among adults in the Appalachian counties of Kentucky, Ohio, and Pennsylvania, where 34.1 percent of the three-state sample reported daily smoking; in Appalachian Kentucky, 40.7 percent of adults reported daily smoking, as did 25.1 percent of Appalachian Ohioans and 33.9 percent of Appalachian Pennsylvanians.[8]

Given the health consequences associated with smoking during pregnancy, the maternal smoking rates in parts of Appalachia (Tennessee, West Virginia, and Kentucky) are concerning. In 2016, 20 to 25 percent of women in the region smoked during pregnancy. Some Appalachian counties have even higher maternal smoking rates. In 2018, two counties in Appalachian Kentucky had maternal smoking rates greater than 40 percent, and in twenty-two counties, the rates exceeded 30 percent.[9]

Published surveillance reports on the use of smokeless tobacco (chewing tobacco, snuff, or snus—a moist tobacco product held between the lips and gums) among all Appalachian adults are limited; however, 2018 BRFSS data indicate that West Virginia leads the nation in smokeless tobacco use among adults, at 6.2 percent versus 2.3 percent (median) nationally. Population-based data from Appalachian counties in Kentucky (2017) suggest that 2.6 percent of adults use smokeless tobacco some days or every day.[10]

Tobacco-use trends among Appalachian youth commonly follow adult trends. For example, in 2017, 14.4 percent of West Virginia high school students reported current cigarette smoking, compared with 8.8 percent of US high school students. One-fourth (25.6 percent) of middle and high school students reported current tobacco use in the Youth Appalachian Tobacco Study (2014–2016), which covered the Appalachian regions of Kentucky, North Carolina, and New York. Owusu and colleagues, using data from 2015–2016, reported that among a sample of Appalachian Tennessee middle school students, 13.2 percent had used alternative tobacco (noncigarette) products at least once, including 5.9 percent who used smokeless tobacco.[11]

Nationally, the use of e-cigarettes and vaping products is on the rise among both youths and adults. As a result, there has been an alarming increase in related health consequences, including lung injuries with acute and chronic effects. Few studies of e-cigarette use among Appalachians have been reported in the literature. Researchers at the University of Kentucky Markey Cancer Center found that 21 percent of Appalachian Kentucky adults (2017) reported using e-cigarettes daily or on some days. A review of 2017 YRBSS data found that states with Appalachian counties generally trend around the national estimate of e-cigarette use among high school students (13.2 percent); the exception was North Carolina, at 22.1 percent. E-cigarettes were the most commonly used alternative tobacco products (at 9.3 percent) among the Appalachian Tennessee youth described in the study by Owusu and colleagues.[12]

Diet, Physical Activity, and Weight

Poor diet and physical inactivity contribute to 15 percent of all deaths, primarily through the clinical manifestation of being overweight (body mass index [BMI] 25.0 to <30.0) and obese (BMI ≥ 30.0) and the link to chronic conditions such as cancer, diabetes, stroke, and heart disease. According to 2012 BRFSS data, nearly one-third (31.0 percent) of Appalachian adults are considered obese, compared with 27.1 percent of their non-Appalachian counterparts and 27.4 percent of all Americans. Similar to the smoking rates described earlier, Appalachian individuals residing in the Central (34.7 percent) and North Central (33.4 percent) subregions have the highest rates of obesity in the region as a whole; additional disparities appear between rural Appalachian individuals (33.1 percent) and those living in large metro areas (29.5 percent) and between economically distressed (34.7 percent) and nondistressed (30.7 percent) counties. Vanderpool and colleagues reported that 68.2 percent of the combined sample of Appalachian Kentuckians, Ohioans, and Pennsylvanians were overweight or obese based on BMI calculations from self-reported height and weight values.[13]

When specifically examining physical activity, more than one-quarter of Appalachians (28.4 percent) reported engaging in no leisure-time physical activity in a typical week, compared with 22.6 percent of non-Appalachian individuals and 23.1 percent of Americans in 2012. Approximately one-third of Appalachian individuals living in Central Appalachia (33.8 percent), rural Appalachia (31.8 percent), and distressed counties (33.9 percent) reported no weekly leisure-time activity.[14]

Research conducted in Appalachian Kentucky among residents recruited from churches and community organizations found that 70 percent of participants were not meeting recommended levels of weekly fruit and vegetable intake and 94 percent were not getting the recommended level of physical activity. Additional disparities were found by age, with younger individuals (aged eighteen to fifty-nine) consuming significantly fewer fruits and vegetables and older individuals (aged sixty and older) reporting significantly less moderate to vigorous physical activity. Paskett and colleagues found that when categorizing overall dietary behaviors (i.e., intake of fruits, vegetables, fish, whole grains, sugar-sweetened beverages [SSBs], and sodium) into poor, intermediate, and ideal levels, 91 percent of survey respondents from Appalachian Ohio fell into the poor or intermediate categories. In addition, 22.3 percent of respondents reported zero days of moderate physical activity per week.[15]

Despite the importance of monitoring and intervening in adolescent obesity and its related health behaviors, there are few published surveillance reports focused on Appalachian youths. Kramer and colleagues estimated the prevalence of county-level adolescent obesity for 2007–2011 and found the highest rates (20.1–41.1 percent quintile) in the Deep South and Central and Southern Appalachia. Based on YRBSS data from 2017, states with Appalachian counties trend higher than the national estimate of obesity among high school students (14.8 percent): for example, 20.2 percent of Kentucky adolescents and 19.5 percent of West Virginia adolescents are obese. In 2015 overweight and obese rates (based on self-reported BMI) among middle school students in southwestern Appalachian Virginia were close to 40 percent. Using data from the 2012 Team Up for Healthy Living trial conducted in regional high schools in Southern Appalachia (Tennessee), Wang and colleagues reported that 19.8 percent of students are overweight and 26.6 percent are obese. Based on data collected in 2006 and 2007, researchers working with an elementary school in southeastern Appalachian Ohio found that 21 percent of the children (aged six to eleven) were overweight. In all three studies, male children and adolescents were more likely to be overweight than females.[16]

Regarding exercise and dietary behaviors among youths in Appalachia, small regional studies have found concerning results, such as a higher consumption of SSBs among children. For example, in 2009–2010 almost half of Appalachian third graders in Ohio consumed at least one SSB daily. Another study conducted among rural high schools in Appalachian Ohio found that participants reported higher SSB consumption levels and lower physical activity levels than adolescents nationally. Data from the 2017 YRBSS show a similar pattern throughout states in the Appalachian region. In Tennessee 10 percent of students reported not eating vegetables during the seven days prior to the survey, versus only 7.2 percent of students nationally. Moreover, almost one-fourth (24.3 percent) of students in South Carolina reported being less physically active (i.e., they "were not physically active for a total of at least 60 minutes on at least one day during the seven days prior to the survey"), compared with 15.4 percent of students nationally.[17]

Health Care Avoidance

Health care avoidance is different from—but sometimes influenced by—access to health care, which is discussed in other chapters. Avoidance of health care may lead to negative health outcomes, including late-stage cancer diagnoses, HIV mortality, and symptoms of heart disease. In addition, delay or avoidance of health care is associated with decreased rates of cancer screening, increased hospital costs, and greater rates of infectious disease transmission.[18]

Broadly, surveillance of health care avoidance among Appalachia's people has been conducted using HINTS data. The primary outcome question read as follows: "Some people avoid visiting their doctor even when they suspect they should. Would you say this is true for you, or not true for you?" Vanderpool and Huang found that 42.4 percent of Appalachian individuals reported that this was true, compared with 35.4 percent of non-Appalachian individuals ($p = 0.0266$). Among those respondents answering "true," additional questions assessed the reasons for avoidance. Although the differences were not statistically significant, more Appalachian individuals than their non-Appalachian counterparts reported feeling uncomfortable having their body examined (38.3 versus 33.4 percent), fearing they had a serious illness (39.3 versus 35.4 percent), and thinking about death (19.0 versus 13.5 percent). Prior qualitative research involving Appalachian Virginians and Tennesseans also provides evidence of health care–avoidant behaviors, specifically related to cancer: "The inability to even think beyond. They are surviving day to day. They don't have time to think about whether they're going to survive five years from now. So, they put off [going to the doctor]. That's just one more trouble they don't need to work with." Other sentiments include: "If I ignore it [cancer], it might go away." In addition to other individual and contextual influences, health care avoidance may play a role in the lower rates of primary and secondary prevention activities such as tobacco cessation, cancer screening (e.g., breast, cervical, lung, colorectal), and human papillomavirus (HPV) vaccination among Appalachia's residents.[19]

Why Are These Behaviors More Prevalent in Appalachia?

Appalachian residents and communities fall well below national public health goals for reducing the prevalence of smoking, obesity, and poor diet and physical inactivity. There are also pointed disparities within Appalachian subregions and specific communities. In addition, data suggest that Appalachians may be more likely to avoid seeking health care services even when they know they need care. The reasons why these health behaviors are more prevalent in Appalachia are complex, multilevel in nature, and inextricably linked to a variety of factors: socioeconomic and demographic disparities, historical and cultural factors, personal preferences and attitudes, environmental and geographic context, experiences with health care professionals and systems, and related policy making at all governmental levels.[20]

Common across all three selected health behaviors is the economic and educational deprivation present in Appalachia, particularly the Central subregion, and its negative influence on residents' health and well-being. In addition, many communities in Appalachia have shortages of health professionals providing primary care, mental health care, specialty care, and dentistry. These shortages impact residents' ability to access prevention, screening, and treatment-related services. Family and peer behavioral norms, particularly related to tobacco use and diet, are also influential in Appalachia. Moreover, states and counties across the region lack policies that are supportive of health and wellness, such as enacting smoke-free legislation, imposing higher sales tax on tobacco products and SSBs, ensuring that US Department of Agriculture nutrition standards are met during and after school hours, requiring dedicated time for physical activity among students, implementing work-site wellness initiatives, expanding Medicaid, and increasing the minimum age to purchase tobacco products.[21]

Specific to tobacco use, the history of tobacco production, sale, and use in Appalachia is a major factor in the region's elevated smoking rates. Many communities are conflicted between supporting local tobacco-growing families (as well as individuals in the community who smoke) and enacting local tobacco control policies. One strategy is to assess readiness and build capacity at the local level; this work has been effective in Appalachian Kentucky, where several counties have passed clean indoor air ordinances. In addition to history, communities must tackle the tobacco industry's targeted marketing of tobacco products in rural areas, particularly among the young. Notably, Tompkins and colleagues found that the majority of Appalachian youths perceive the policy of increasing the minimum age to purchase tobacco products to twenty-one to be ineffective in decreasing tobacco use. Liu and colleagues also noted differences in the perception of the relative safety of smokeless tobacco versus cigarettes among adolescents and adults in Appalachian Ohio.[22]

Environmental context also plays a role in shaping health disparities across Appalachia. Included here are factors such as food insecurity, food deserts, and food affordability, which jointly contribute to the region's higher prevalence of poor diet, physical inactivity, and elevated obesity rates. Notably, there are 14 percent fewer grocery stores per 1,000 population in Appalachia than in the United States as a whole. Booth and colleagues identified a significant relationship between rising county-level obesity rates and the decreasing number of grocery stores per capita within the Appalachian region. Related to this, there may be fewer facilities dedicated to physical activity and limited areas where it is safe to exercise due to poor road and weather conditions. There have also been decreases in farming, gardening, and canning (of homegrown produce) across many rural and Appalachian communities, although farm-to-table initiatives, cooperative extension collaborations, and farmers' markets have seen renewed growth in the past decade. In considering health-related perceptions, Rice and colleagues—using HINTS data—found that Appalachian individuals are less likely than non-Appalachian individuals to believe that lifestyle factors are related to obesity.[23]

Health care avoidance may stem from beliefs about health and disease, including perceptions about the preventability of disease, prevention recommendations, causes of disease, survivability, self-efficacy, and fatalism. For example, Vanderpool and colleagues reported that 71 percent of Appalachian Kentuckians agreed that "everything" causes cancer, compared with 63 percent of Appalachian Ohioans and 57 percent of Appalachian Pennsylvanians ($p = 0.001$). In addition, 81 percent of respondents from Appalachian Kentucky indicated agreement with the statement that there are too many cancer prevention recommendations to know which ones to follow, compared with 61 percent of Appalachian Ohioans and 74 percent of Appalachian Pennsylvanians ($p = 0.020$). Close to three-fourths (72 percent) of Appalachian Kentuckians reported that when they think of cancer, they automatically think of death; this response was notably lower among Appalachian Ohioans (55 percent) and Appalachian Pennsylvanians (57 percent).[24]

Other locally conducted research has found that fatalistic beliefs among individuals and communities can deter health care utilization, such as completing the HPV vaccination series and having a Pap test among women in Appalachian Kentucky. In addition, Hutson and colleagues, in their poignantly titled paper "The Mountains Hold Things In," describe Appalachian Virginians' and Tennesseans' perceptions of storytelling (cancer stories are trapped in the mountains), cancer collectivism (cancer affects all families and is everywhere), problems with the health care system (access, trust, navigation, perceptions of invisibility), and cancer expectations (they would rather not know) as influencing residents' interactions—and lack thereof—with cancer-related health care services.[25]

Evidence-Based Programs

Evidence-based health programs and practices are developed through the study of existing high-quality, reproducible research. Such studies have applied program planning frameworks, engaged the community in assessment, and conducted thorough evaluations to provide results that guide and inform the selection of programs, policies, and practices to improve health. For successful implementation, evidence-based programs must be balanced with the population's needs and preferences, resources—including the availability of personnel with the required skills—and the environmental and organizational context.[26]

As described throughout this chapter, tobacco use, poor diet, physical inactivity, and health care avoidance are prevalent in Appalachia, resulting in numerous adverse health outcomes. The environmental context includes geographically isolated populations, low socioeconomic status, limited policies supportive of health, long-standing behavioral and social norms, and limited public health infrastructure and access to clinical services. Communities often begin the process of identifying how best to deal with these challenges by forming coalitions and task forces of concerned residents. Although this demonstrates local support for interventions and programs to address extant health disparities, it can result in failure if the strategies developed to solve the problem are not grounded in evidence. Political pressure, media campaigns, anecdotal evidence, and long-used or traditional approaches often influence the strategies chosen by these groups to address specific health concerns. In addition, there may be no formal evaluation plan to measure and address variations in the program's implementation, outcome, and impact on the targeted community. In Appalachia, suggestions that such groups follow the evidence base to inform individual- and community-level behavioral interventions are often described as "overwhelming" and "restrictive," thus affecting decision makers' willingness to use evidence-based programs.[27]

Researchers recognize the importance of cultural adaptation of evidence-based programs to accommodate the needs of those populations most affected by health disparities. However, not all populations, settings, or health issues can be addressed by existing evidence-based programs; specifically, evidence-based programs developed or adapted for Appalachian populations are scarce. To increase the participation in and success of any initiative designed to improve health behaviors in Appalachian populations, several elements are needed: adaptation of evidence-based programs to leverage the strong sense of self-reliance, family and social networks, faith, storytelling traditions, social capital, and importance of place among the Appalachian people; reduction of structural barriers; and growth in individual and community self-efficacy.[28]

The following evidence-based, Appalachia-centric public health programs serve as tangible examples of community members, health care professionals, and researchers committed to reducing disparities in tobacco use; diet, physical activity, and weight; and health care avoidance. They illustrate partnerships with the faith community, lay health advisers, health care professionals, hospitals, federally qualified health centers (FQHCs), work sites, and schools. In addition, the programs work at multiple levels of influence (provider, patient, community) and with different populations (pregnant women, youths, adults).

Tobacco

Faith Moves Mountains

Using a faith-based model, this randomized controlled trial of a community-based smoking cessation intervention included six rural Appalachian Kentucky counties. It utilized the twelve-week Cooper/Clayton method to stop smoking; the program's orientation, based on social support, made it particularly applicable to a population that values social connections. Participants met weekly with lay health advisers, received didactic information, took part in group interactions, and received nicotine replacement therapy. The nicotine replacement therapy was provided at no charge, thus removing the barrier of cost for low-income or underinsured participants. At the end of the study, participants from the intervention group of churches had 13.6 times better odds of self-reported quitting than participants from the control group of churches.[29]

Smoking Cessation Program for Pregnant and Postpartum Women in West Virginia

The Health Education for Prenatal Providers in Appalachia (HEPPA) program was developed to address health disparities and limited prenatal health resources among at-risk women in four counties in West Virginia. Women in these areas often have to travel outside their county of residence to access prenatal care. Based on the office-based smoking cessation model of the American College of Obstetricians and Gynecologists, HEPPA focused on increasing health care and social services providers' knowledge of prenatal smoking cessation strategies. Participants attended a 1.5-hour training session, which used an interdisciplinary team approach to cover the five As of smoking cessation counseling: *asking* about tobacco use, *advising* on how to quit, *assessing* the patient's willingness to quit, *assisting* with a quit attempt, and *arranging* follow-up with the patient. More than 90 percent of participants rated the program's quality and content positively (good, very good, or excellent). HEPPA's evaluation indicated its effectiveness in increasing discussions about smoking cessation between providers and pregnant women. More specifically, there were significant increases in discussions about the *advising* ($p = 0.015$) and *assisting* ($p = 0.007$) steps of the counseling program.[30]

Spit It Out–West Virginia

The Southern Coalfields Regional Tobacco Prevention Network Office implemented Spit It Out–West Virginia to address the high rates of smokeless tobacco use in that state. The program included creative, culturally appropriate advertising via billboards and radio ads to educate residents about the adverse effects of smokeless tobacco. Spit It Out–West Virginia engaged the faith-based community to encourage tobacco cessation and the business community to distribute materials about the program. It also held community events to educate the public, and targeted workshops on tobacco cessation were conducted in specific workplaces.

In addition to reaching individuals via workshops and counseling, Spit It Out–West Virginia awarded grants to faith-based institutions to organize educational events on tobacco cessation and the dangers of smokeless tobacco. During the first year of the program, five businesses adopted tobacco-free workplace policies, and county-level tobacco cessation enrollment through a hotline increased by 800 percent.[31]

Smoke-Free Policies in Rural Kentucky

Smoke-free policies have a positive impact on population health, such as improvements in various health outcomes among hospitality workers and fewer hospitalizations for asthma and acute coronary events. Given this evidence, researchers have examined various aspects of planning and implementing smoke-free policies in rural communities throughout Appalachian Kentucky, including an assessment of community readiness. For instance, Hahn and colleagues gauged community readiness for smoke-free policies in thirty rural Kentucky counties, many of which produced tobacco. Elected officials and community stakeholders from these counties were interviewed and were asked questions about several important elements of community readiness (e.g., community resources, community activities to increase knowledge about the effects of secondhand smoke, and community leadership). These interview findings, along with an evaluation of county-level tobacco control efforts, were used to determine the level of readiness. Overall, counties with higher adult smoking rates and higher levels of tobacco production were less ready to implement smoke-free policies ($p = 0.004$ and $p = 0.002$, respectively), regardless of the strength of the tobacco control measures enacted. Another study assessed the impact of local-level smoke-free regulations on smoking rates in Kentucky counties. Those findings suggest that smoking prevalence rates are lower (5 to 6 percent) in counties that have enacted smoke-free ordinances ($p < 0.001$). There also appears to be a small dose-response relationship between smoking rates and the level of smoke-free ordinance enacted (i.e., none, weak/moderate, comprehensive).[32]

Physical Activity and Nutrition

Walk by Faith

This faith-based study randomly assigned participants in five Appalachian states (Ohio, Kentucky, Pennsylvania, West Virginia, and Virginia) to a monthly diet and exercise educational session (Walk by Faith) or a cancer screening and education program (Ribbons of Faith). Churches were selected as key partners in this study due to the importance of faith-based organizations in Appalachian communities. Both interventions were originally developed by Appalachian community coalitions in Ohio and included local navigators from the churches to promote and deliver programming. Walk by Faith included the identification of safe walking paths and organized walking groups, and Ribbons of Faith promoted cancer education and encouraged age-appropriate cancer screening. The primary outcome was weight loss, mainly in male participants, from baseline to twelve months. The study noted that Walk by Faith participants experienced a relative weight loss of 1.4 percent compared with Ribbons of Faith participants, and increasing levels of participation in the program correlated with greater weight loss ($p = 0.002$).[33]

Trinity Hospital Twin City Fit for Life

The original Fit for Life (FFL) program, created in 2003 in Appalachian Ohio, included a twelve-week wellness and disease prevention program for adult men and women. Each ninety-minute session covered a variety of health improvement topics delivered by physicians, chiropractors, wellness educators, and other health professionals. The FFL program's goal was to reduce obesity rates among participants by teaching them the elements of a healthy lifestyle. Topics included stress management, nutrition for life, food labels, and cardiovascular fitness.[34]

In 2012 FFL was expanded and replicated in east-central Ohio and four bordering Appalachian counties. The goal was to implement the program on a larger scale using a train-the-trainer approach. From 2013 to 2015 participants who completed the program reported an average weight loss of 2.7 kilograms (5.95 pounds), with more than half reporting a loss of at least 3 percent of body weight; nearly 70 percent of participants reported increased physical activity per week. In addition, participants reported eating more fruits and vegetables (67 percent improvement) and whole grains (54 percent) and less trans fats (54 percent) and high-fructose corn syrup (59 percent). FFL subsequently received funding from the federal Office of Rural Health Policy to expand the program into diabetes prevention (2015–2018).[35]

Sodabriety

Community-based participatory research conducted in Pike County, Ohio, identified young people's consumption of SSBs as a health concern. Sodabriety, a thirty-day student-led intervention, was launched to reduce SSB consumption among teenagers. High school students designed commercials, T-shirts, and flyers and recorded information about SSBs, including vending machine choices, to inspire other students to participate in the challenge to reduce their consumption of SSBs. During the challenge, students were encouraged to drink water, unsweetened tea, or diet soda and to record their consumption of SSBs immediately after the thirty-day challenge and thirty days post intervention. Immediately following the Sodabriety intervention, student logs indicated that their average SSB consumption decreased from 2.32 to 1.32 per day ($p < 0.001$) and from 4.30 to 2.64 per week ($p < 0.001$); water consumption increased by 19 percent. Sodabriety was later expanded to high schools in Tennessee.[36]

Plate It Up Kentucky Proud

To improve physical activity levels and the intake of healthy foods in rural Kentucky, researchers at the University of Kentucky collaborated with family and consumer science extension agents and the Kentucky Department of Agriculture to implement a community-level intervention in six counties, five of them in Appalachian Kentucky. The intervention involved a social marketing campaign called Plate It Up Kentucky Proud (PIU). The campaign involved supermarket-based elements, including healthy food samples, grocery cart placards with recipes using in-season fruits and vegetables, and PIU banners outside each store. Farmers' markets also participated in PIU and used incentives, such as gas cards, to encourage community members to shop there. Participating counties encouraged physical activity through the improvement of community resources, such as the installation of walking trails and water-bottle filling stations in existing parks. County extension agents then held events to promote the use of these newly enhanced resources. The PIU social marketing campaign was evaluated by surveying county residents in years 1 and 2 about their fruit and vegetable intake, physical activity levels, and grocery shopping behaviors. Results revealed increases in the mean number of servings per day of both fruits (2.71 to 2.94) and vegetables (2.54 to 2.72); there was also an increase in those who shopped at farmers' markets once a week (from 7 percent to 12 percent).[37]

Health Care Avoidance

As described earlier, health care avoidance is complex and can be influenced by many factors. One approach to bringing about positive change among Appalachians is to make interacting with the health care system easier and more streamlined, to address barriers to care, and to make care more affordable, particularly for preventive health services.

Proactive Office Encounter

Kaiser Permanente in Southern California originally developed the Proactive Office Encounter (POE) to identify preventive care gaps among its primary care patient population. POE provides a systematic approach for clinical settings to ensure that patients are up to date on preventive care services such as cancer screenings, obesity prevention, tobacco cessation, immunizations, medication management, and diabetes care.[38]

POE strategically uses information technology, new workflows, and continuous quality development techniques to assess patients' compliance with preventive care guidelines appropriate for their age and health status *at each visit*, regardless of the reason for the visit (whether for chronic disease maintenance or acute illness). In the year following POE's adaptation and implementation in an eight-site FQHC serving five counties in Appalachian Kentucky, there were significant increases in colorectal cancer screenings (36 percent), as well as more than five times the number of HIV screenings (831 to 4,371) and eight times the number of hepatitis C screenings (378 to 3,334). In addition, the implementation of POE decreased the need for patients to return to the clinic for separate wellness appointments, thereby alleviating cost- and transportation-related barriers. The intervention also improved patient-provider communication and facilitated shared decision making, as providers introduced patient-centered, prevention-oriented health care at every encounter with the health care system.[39]

The Health Wagon

The Health Wagon is a mobile medical clinic that provides free health care, including acute and chronic disease management, laboratory and diagnostic services, medication assistance, and dental and eye care, to Appalachian populations. In addition, the mobile clinic offers specialty consultations, diabetes supplies, and prescription medications at no cost to participants. Most patients seen by the Health Wagon are uninsured, and they present for the treatment of a variety of issues, including hypertension, diabetes, and depression.[40]

The Health Wagon delivered more than $5.6 million worth of health care services to rural communities in Appalachian Virginia in 2018, and it has increased its patient population over time. In 2009 the Health Wagon served 2,900 patients, resulting in 3,165 patient encounters; in 2018 more than 4,700 patients were served, with 16,670 patient encounters. Services are provided through collaboration among multiple organizational partners, including the University of Virginia Health System and hospital laboratories in the area. In addition, partners such as the Appalachian College of Pharmacy provide educational materials for participants. The Health Wagon helps break down both financial and access barriers to health care in rural Central Appalachia.[41]

Kentucky Homeplace

Kentucky Homeplace (KH) is an initiative led by the University of Kentucky Center of Excellence in Rural Health to address health disparities in Appalachian Kentucky. When the initiative began in 1994, it served only one town in eastern Kentucky; it has since grown to serve residents in thirty counties in Appalachian Kentucky. KH focuses on training and utilizing community health workers (CHWs) to provide health-related services in the communities where they reside. These services are free of charge and can be provided in patients' homes; they include preventive care such as coaching on healthy lifestyle choices, coordination of immunizations and cancer screenings, tobacco cessation education, and implementation of chronic disease self-management programs. KH served almost 162,000 clients from July 2001 to June 2018 and provided more than 4.9 million services. The initiative has proved to be effective in various ways. For example, a return-on-investment analysis determined that for every dollar invested in KH, $11.20 is saved. In addition, KH interventions have resulted in improvements in client awareness and action related to health behaviors, including lung and colorectal cancer screening and self-management of diabetes. For example, Feltner and colleagues conducted a study involving a KH program led by CHWs aimed at improving awareness and knowledge of colorectal cancer screening options. Participants' mean score measuring colorectal cancer–related knowledge increased from 4.27 before the program to 4.57 after it ($p < 0.001$); in addition, more participants asked their health care providers about colorectal cancer screening (increasing from 27.6 percent to 34.1 percent).[42]

Additional Evidence-Based Strategies

Additional strategies to address health care avoidance may include individual-, provider-, and community-level communication and education initiatives—developed in collaboration with Appalachian residents—that present evidence-based guidelines in an understandable, culturally relevant manner so that individuals feel confident and empowered to follow recommendations that may save their lives. Suggestions for the future include the dissemination of low-literacy-level visual or audio educational materials and messaging through community- and faith-based initiatives; improved access to online health information and technology infrastructure; explanation of local health statistics, including incidence, mortality, and survival, in lay terms to further the public's understanding; passage of supportive health policies at state and local levels; and the creation of positive social norms to help alleviate the health-related fear, stigma, and confusion commonly observed in Appalachian populations.[43]

Sources of Evidence-Based Strategies and Interventions

Before developing a new health improvement initiative, public health practitioners, health care providers, and community organizers are strongly encouraged to review evidence-based or evidence-informed practices for information about what has already been studied and proved to work for a specific health condition (e.g., cancer, cardiovascular disease, diabetes, mental health) or in a specific setting (e.g., urban, rural, hospital, school). The following are sources of evidence-based interventions and programming:

- *Guide to Community Preventive Services* (also known as "The Community Guide")—The Community Preventive Service Task Force (CPSTF) uses a science-based approach to review a wide range of health topics and interventions to identify those with sufficient (or insufficient) evidence.[a]
- *Rural Health Information Hub (RHIhub)*—Funded by the federal Office of Rural Health Policy, RHIhub provides online access to

planning and development tools and other learning resources related to rural health needs and opportunities to address them.[b]

- **Robert Wood Johnson Foundation (RWJF)**—The guiding principles of the RWJF include implementing lasting change based on the best available evidence. The foundation provides information on research, evaluation, and learning in the areas of health systems, healthy communities, healthy children and families, and leadership for better health. The RWJF is committed to collaborating to build a national culture of health that gives everyone the opportunity to live a healthier life.[c]

- **County Health Rankings & Roadmaps**—This program, which is funded by the RWJF, includes What Works for Health, which rates the effectiveness of policies, programs, systems, and environmental strategies that can affect health.[d]

- **Cancer Control P.L.A.N.E.T.**—Sponsored by the National Cancer Institute (NCI), Centers for Disease Control and Prevention (CDC), Agency for Healthcare Research and Quality (AHRQ), and International Cancer Control Partnership, Cancer Control P.L.A.N.E.T. (Plan, Link, Act, Network with Evidence-based Tools) provides data and other resources to planners, researchers, and program staff for the design, implementation, and evaluation of evidence-based cancer control programs. Its Evidence-Based Cancer Control Programs (EBCCP) database is a source of cancer control interventions.[e]

- **Agency for Healthcare Research and Quality (AHRQ)**—The AHRQ's goal is to improve the safety, quality, accessibility, and affordability of health care. It works with partners to ensure that evidence is both understood and used. The AHRQ website includes a Clinical Guidelines and Recommendations page where users can connect to information from the US Preventive Services Task Force on evidence-based prevention guidelines.[f]

- **Cochrane Library**—Cochrane provides systematic reviews and other synthesized research information to promote evidence-informed decision making on health.[g]

- **National Center for Chronic Disease Prevention and Health Promotion (NCCDPHP)**—Through its "Success Stories," the NCCDPHP identifies how communities are using CDC funding to create healthy environments.[h]

- **Substance Abuse and Mental Health Services Administration (SAMHSA)**—SAMHSA's Evidence-Based Practices Resource Center provides evidence-based information and tools to communities and those working in clinical settings.[i]

a. US Department of Health and Human Services, "The Community Guide," https://www.thecommunityguide.org/.
b. Rural Health Information Hub (RHIhub), https://www.ruralhealthinfo.org/.
c. Robert Wood Johnson Foundation, https://www.rwjf.org/.
d. County Health Rankings & Roadmaps, https://www.countyhealthrankings.org/.
e. NCI, Cancer Control P.L.A.N.E.T., https://cancercontrolplanet.cancer.gov/planet/.
f. US Department of Health and Human Services, Agency for Healthcare Research and Quality, https://www.ahrq.gov/.
g. Cochrane Library, https://www.cochranelibrary.com/.
h. CDC, "National Center for Chronic Disease Prevention and Health Promotion (NCCDPHP)—Success Stories," August 8, 2019, https://www.cdc.gov/chronicdisease/programs-impact/success-stories/index.htm.
i. US Department of Health and Human Services, Substance Abuse and Mental Health Services Administration (SAMHSA)—Evidence-Based Practices Resource Center, https://www.samhsa.gov/ebp-resource-center.

Several modifiable health behaviors that are prevalent among Appalachian residents contribute to the leading causes of disease morbidity and mortality in the region. The key message is that these behaviors can be prevented, changed, improved, enhanced, and terminated. Indeed, tobacco cessation, healthy diets and physical activity, and engagement with health care professionals can all be achieved through the implementation of evidence-based programs and interventions conducted in collaboration with Appalachian communities and key stakeholders. Importantly, these evidence-based strategies and interventions are also effective in addressing many other health behaviors that were not discussed in this chapter but are prominent across Appalachia.

Notes

Robin C. Vanderpool and Kelly D. Blake participated in the writing of this chapter as part of their official duties as National Institutes of Health (NIH) employees, and their contribution is considered a work of the US government.

1. Sherry Murphy, Jiaquan Xu, Kenneth Kochanek, and Elizabeth Arias, *Mortality in the United States, 2017* (Washington, DC: Centers for Disease Control and Prevention, 2018), https://www.cdc.gov/nchs/products/databriefs/db328.htm; Julie L. Marshall et al., *Health*

Disparities in Appalachia (Washington, DC: Appalachian Regional Commission, 2017), https://www.arc.gov/assets/research_reports/Health_Disparities_in_Appalachia _August_2017.pdf; Sharon Rodriguez, Nathan Vanderford, Bin Huang, and Robin Vanderpool, "A Social-Ecological Review of Cancer Disparities in Kentucky," *Southern Medical Journal* 111, no. 4 (2018): 213–19; Ali Mokdad et al., "Trends and Patterns of Disparities in Cancer Mortality among US Counties, 1980–2014," *JAMA* 317, no. 4 (2017): 388–406; Michael Meit, Megan Heffernan, Erin Tanenbaum, and Topher Hoffman, *Appalachian Diseases of Despair* (Washington, DC: Appalachian Regional Commission, 2017), https://www.arc.gov/assets /research_reports/appalachiandiseasesofdespairaugust2017.pdf; Kate Beatty et al., *Health Disparities Related to Obesity in Appalachia: Practical Strategies and Recommendations for Communities* (Washington, DC: Appalachian Regional Commission, 2019), https://www.arc .gov/assets/research_reports/HealthDisparitiesRelatedtoObesityinAppalachiaApr2019.pdf; East Tennessee State University and NORC at the University of Chicago, *Health Disparities Related to Smoking in Appalachia: Practical Strategies and Recommendations for Communities* (Washington, DC: Appalachian Regional Commission, 2019), https://www.arc.gov/assets /research_reports/HealthDispairitiesRelatedtoSmokinginAppalachiaApr2019.pdf.

2. J. McGinnis and William Foege, "Actual Causes of Death in the United States," *JAMA* 270, no. 18 (1993): 2207–12; Ali Mokdad, James Marks, Donna Stroup, and Julie Gerberding, "Actual Causes of Death in the United States, 2000," *JAMA* 291, no. 10 (2004): 1238–45.

3. McGinnis and Foege, "Actual Causes of Death"; Mokdad et al., "Actual Causes of Death"; Sharon Byrne, "Healthcare Avoidance: A Critical Review," *Holistic Nursing Practice* 22, no. 5 (2008): 280–92; Karen Glanz, Barbara Rimer, and K. Viswanath, eds., *Health Behavior: Theory, Research, and Practice,* 5th ed. (San Francisco: Jossey-Bass, 2015); Vicki Freimuth, Judith Stein, and Thomas Kean, *Searching for Health Information: The Cancer Information Service Model* (Philadelphia: University of Pennsylvania Press, 1989); Marvin Zuckerman, "Sensation Seeking and Behavior Disorders," *Archives of General Psychiatry* 45, no. 5 (1988): 502–4; Anne Case and Angus Deaton, "Rising Morbidity and Mortality in Midlife among White Non-Hispanic Americans in the 21st Century," *Proceedings of the National Academy of Sciences of the United States of America* 112, no. 49 (2015): 15078–83; Tom Farley and Deborah Cohen, *Prescription for a Healthy Nation: A New Approach to Improving Our Lives by Fixing Our Everyday World* (Boston: Beacon Press, 2006), 18.

4. Marshall et al., *Health Disparities in Appalachia;* Beatty et al., *Health Disparities Related to Obesity;* East Tennessee State University and NORC, *Health Disparities Related to Smoking;* Sadie Hutson, Kelly Dorgan, Amber Phillips, and Bruce Behringer, "The Mountains Hold Things In: The Use of Community Research Review Work Groups to Address Cancer Disparities in Appalachia," *Oncology Nursing Forum* 34, no. 6 (2007): 1133–39; Angela Spleen, Eugene Lengerich, Fabian Camacho, and Robin Vanderpool, "Health Care Avoidance among Rural Populations: Results from a Nationally Representative Survey," *Journal of Rural Health* 30, no. 1 (2014): 79–88; Robin Vanderpool, "Kentucky Tobacco Users' Calls to a National Quitline," *Kentucky Journal of Communication* 27, no. 2 (2008): 171–78; Lila Finey Rutten et al., "Use of E-Cigarettes among Current Smokers: Associations among Reasons for Use, Quit Intentions, and Current Tobacco Use," *Nicotine & Tobacco Research* 17, no. 10 (2015): 1228–34; Elise Rice et al., "Beliefs about Behavioral Determinants of Obesity in Appalachia, 2011–2014," *Public Health Reports* 133, no. 4 (2018): 379–84; Chan Thai et al., "'Keep It Realistic': Reactions to and Recommendations for Physical Activity Promotion Messages from Focus Groups of Women," *American Journal of Health*

Promotion 33, no. 6 (2019): 903–11; Robin Vanderpool and Bin Huang, "Cancer Risk Perceptions, Beliefs, and Physician Avoidance in Appalachia: Results from the 2008 HINTS Survey," *Journal of Health Communication* 15, suppl. 3 (2010): 78–91; Robin Vanderpool et al., "Adaptation of an Evidence-Based Intervention to Improve Preventive Care Practices in a Federally Qualified Health Center in Appalachian Kentucky," *Journal of Health Care for the Poor and Underserved* 27, no. 4A (2016): 46–52.

5. Whitney Zahnd et al., "Challenges of Using Nationally Representative, Population-Based Surveys to Assess Rural Cancer Disparities," *Preventive Medicine* 129S (2019): 105812; Robin Vanderpool et al., "Adapting and Implementing Evidence-Based Cancer Education Interventions in Rural Appalachia: Real World Experiences and Challenges," *Rural and Remote Health* 11, no. 4 (2011):1807; Beatty et al., *Health Disparities Related to Obesity;* East Tennessee State University and NORC, *Health Disparities Related to Smoking;* Paul Reiter, Mira Katz, and Electra Paskett, "HPV Vaccination among Adolescent Females from Appalachia: Implications for Cervical Cancer Disparities," *Cancer Epidemiology, Biomarkers, and Prevention* 21, no. 12 (2012): 2220–30.

6. CDC, "Behavioral Risk Factor Surveillance System," 2019, https://www.cdc.gov/brfss/index.html; CDC, "Adolescent and School Health: YRBSS," August 20, 2020, https://www.cdc.gov/healthyyouth/data/yrbs/index.htm; CDC, "National Health Interview Survey," September 9, 2020, https://www.cdc.gov/nchs/nhis/index.htm; NCI, "HINTS," 2019, https://hints.cancer.gov/.

7. Marshall et al., *Health Disparities in Appalachia;* Rice et al., "Beliefs about Behavioral Determinants of Obesity"; Vanderpool and Huang, "Cancer Risk Perceptions"; Reiter et al., "HPV Vaccination among Adolescent Females"; Jennifer Lobo et al., "Disparities in the Use of Diabetes Screening in Appalachia," *Journal of Rural Health* 34, no. 2 (2018): 173–81; ARC, "Counties in Appalachia," https://www.arc.gov/appalachian_region/Countiesin Appalachia.asp; Kelly Blake and Robert Croyle, "Rurality, Rural Identity, and Cancer Control: Evidence from NCI's Population Health Assessment in Cancer Center Catchment Areas Initiative," *Journal of Rural Health* 35, no. 2 (2019): 141–43; Robin Vanderpool et al., "Cancer-Related Beliefs and Perceptions in Appalachia: Findings from 3 States," *Journal of Rural Health* 35, no. 2 (2019): 176–88; Electra Paskett et al., "The CITIES Project: Understanding the Health of Underrepresented Populations in Ohio," *Cancer Epidemiology, Biomarkers, and Prevention* 28, no. 3 (2019): 442–54; Electra Paskett et al., "Correlates of Rural, Appalachian, and Community Identity in the CITIES Cohort," *Journal of Rural Health* 35, no. 2 (2019): 167–75; Lindsay Tompkins et al., "'If You Are Old Enough to Die for Your Country, You Should Be Able to Get a Pinch of Snuff': Views of Tobacco 21 among Appalachian Youth," *Journal of Applied Research on Children* 8, no. 2 (2017): 2; Daniel Owusu et al., "Intention to Try Tobacco among Middle School Students in a Predominantly Rural Environment of Central Appalachia," *Substance Use & Misuse* 54, no. 3 (2019): 449–58; Cilgy Abraham et al., "Factors Influencing Cardiovascular Risk Factors and Health Perception among Kentuckians Living in Appalachia," *Journal of Cardiovascular Nursing* 35, no. 3 (2020): E1–8; Robin Vanderpool, Emily Van Meter Dressler, Lindsay Stradtman, and Richard Crosby, "Fatalistic Beliefs and Completion of the HPV Vaccination Series among a Sample of Young Appalachian Kentucky Women," *Journal of Rural Health* 31, no. 2 (2015): 199–205; Aasha Hoogland, Charles Hoogland, Shoshana Bardach, Yalena Tarasenko, and Nancy Schoenberg, "Health Behaviors in Rural Appalachia," *Southern Medical Journal* 112, no. 8 (2019): 444–49.

8. East Tennessee State University and NORC, *Health Disparities Related to Smoking;* CDC, "Health Effects of Cigarette Smoking," January 17, 2018, https://www.cdc.gov/tobacco

/data_statistics/fact_sheets/health_effects/effects_cig_smoking/index.htm; US Department of Health and Human Services, "Healthy People 2020: Tobacco Use Objectives," 2014, https://www.healthypeople.gov/2020/topics-objectives/topic/tobacco-use/objectives; Marshall et al., *Health Disparities in Appalachia;* CDC, "BRFSS Prevalence & Trends Data," September 13, 2017, https://www.cdc.gov/brfss/brfssprevalence; Vanderpool et al., "Cancer-Related Beliefs."

9. Rural Health Information Hub (RHIhub), https://www.ruralhealthinfo.org/; Patrick Drake, Anne Driscoll, and T. J. Mathews, "Cigarette Smoking during Pregnancy: United States, 2016," CDC, February 2018, https://www.cdc.gov/nchs/products/databriefs/db305 .htm; Kentucky Youth Advocates, "2018 Kentucky KIDS Count County Data Book," 2018, https://kyyouth.org/wp-content/uploads/2018/11/2018_CountyDataBook.pdf.

10. CDC, "BRFSS Prevalence & Trends Data"; Mark Evers, "Administrative Supplements for NCI-Designated Cancer Centers to Support Population Health Assessment in Cancer Center Catchment Areas," National Institutes of Health, National Cancer Institute, 2016.

11. CDC, "2017 High School Youth Risk Behavior Survey Data," 2017, http://nccd.cdc .gov/youthonline/; Tompkins et al., "If You Are Old Enough"; Owusu et al., "Intention to Try Tobacco."

12. US Department of Health and Human Services, "E-Cigarette Use among Youth and Young Adults: A Report of the Surgeon General," 2016, https://e-cigarettes.surgeongen-eral.gov/documents/2016_sgr_full_report_non-508.pdf; Charlotte Schoenborn and Renee Gindi, "Electronic Cigarette Use among Adults: United States, 2014," *NCHS Data Brief* 217 (2015): 1–8; Isaac Ghinai et al., "E-Cigarette Product Use, or Vaping, among Persons with Associated Lung Injury—Illinois and Wisconsin, April–September 2019," *MMWR Morbidity and Mortality Weekly Report* 68, no. 39 (2019): 865–69; CDC, "Outbreak of Lung Injury Associated with E-Cigarette Use, or Vaping," 2019, https://www.cdc.gov/tobacco/basic _information/e-cigarettes/severe-lung-disease.html; Evers, "Administrative Supplements"; CDC, "2017 High School Youth Risk"; Owusu et al., "Intention to Try Tobacco."

13. CDC, "Adult Obesity Causes & Consequences," 2017, https://www.cdc.gov /obesity/adult/causes.html; Marshall et al., *Health Disparities in Appalachia;* Vanderpool et al., "Cancer-Related Beliefs."

14. Marshall et al., *Health Disparities in Appalachia.*

15. Hoogland et al., "Health Behaviors in Rural Appalachia"; Paskett et al., "CITIES Project."

16. CDC, "Child & Teen Healthy Weight and Obesity," 2019, https://www.cdc.gov /nccdphp/dnpao/resources/child-teen-resources.html; Michael Kramer et al., "Geography of Adolescent Obesity in the U.S., 2007–2011," *American Journal of Preventive Medicine* 51, no. 6 (2016): 898–909; CDC, "2017 High School Youth Risk"; Georgianna Mann and Elena Serrano, "The Association between Weight Perception and Weight Intention in Middle School Appalachian Students," *Public Health* 171 (2019): 135–38; Liang Wang et al., "Prevalence of and Risk Factors for Adolescent Obesity in Southern Appalachia, 2012," *Preventing Chronic Disease* 11 (2014): E222; Karen Montgomery-Reagan et al., "Prevalence and Correlates of High Body Mass Index in Rural Appalachian Children Aged 6–11 Years," *Rural and Remote Health* 9, no. 4 (2009): 1234.

17. Laureen Smith and Christopher Holloman, "Piloting 'Sodabriety': A School-Based Intervention to Impact Sugar-Sweetened Beverage Consumption in Rural Appalachian High Schools," *Journal of School Health* 84, no. 3 (2014): 177–84; Laureen Smith, Devin

Laurent, Erica Baumker, and Rick Petosa, "Rates of Obesity and Obesogenic Behaviors of Rural Appalachian Adolescents: How Do They Compare to Other Adolescents or Recommendations?" *Journal of Physical Activity & Health* 15, no. 11 (2018): 874–81; CDC, "2017 High School Youth Risk."

18. Hutson et al., "Mountains Hold Things In"; Spleen et al., "Health Care Avoidance among Rural Populations"; Michael Ohl et al., "Rural Residence Is Associated with Delayed Care Entry and Increased Mortality among Veterans with Human Immunodeficiency Virus Infection," *Medical Care* 48, no. 12 (2010): 1064–70; Noreen Facione, Christine Miaskowski, Marylin Dodd, and Steven Paul, "The Self-Reported Likelihood of Patient Delay in Breast Cancer: New Thoughts for Early Detection," *Preventive Medicine* 34, no. 4 (2002): 397–407; Nancy Altice and Elizabeth Madigan, "Factors Associated with Delayed Care-Seeking in Hospitalized Patients with Heart Failure," *Heart & Lung: The Journal of Critical Care* 41, no. 3 (2012): 244–54; Byrne, "Healthcare Avoidance"; Aleli Kraft et al., "The Health and Cost Impact of Care Delay and the Experimental Impact of Insurance on Reducing Delays," *Journal of Pediatrics* 155, no. 2 (2009): 281–85.e1; Catherine Mercer et al., "How Much Do Delayed Healthcare Seeking, Delayed Care Provision, and Diversion from Primary Care Contribute to the Transmission of STIs?" *Sexually Transmitted Infections* 83, no. 5 (2007): 400–405.

19. Vanderpool and Huang, "Cancer Risk Perceptions"; Hutson et al., "Mountains Hold Things In"; Reiter et al., "HPV Vaccination among Adolescent Females"; Paul Reiter, Alvin Wee, Amy Lehman, and Electra Paskett, "Oral Cancer Screening and Dental Care Use among Women from Ohio Appalachia," *Rural and Remote Health* 12 (2012): 2184; Mira Katz et al., "Adherence to Multiple Cancer Screening Tests among Women Living in Appalachia Ohio," *Cancer Epidemiology, Biomarkers, and Prevention* 24, no. 10 (2015): 1489–94; Nengliano Yao, Hector Alcalá, Roger Anderson, and Rajesh Balkrishnan, "Cancer Disparities in Rural Appalachia: Incidence, Early Detection, and Survivorship," *Journal of Rural Health* 33, no. 4 (2017): 375–81.

20. Rodriguez et al., "Social-Ecological Review of Cancer Disparities"; Beatty et al., *Health Disparities Related to Obesity;* East Tennessee State University and NORC, *Health Disparities Related to Smoking;* Bruce Behringer and Gilbert Friedell, "Appalachia: Where Place Matters in Health," *Preventing Chronic Disease* 3, no. 4 (2006): A113; Richard Couto, Nancy Simpson, and Gale Harris, eds., *Sowing Seeds in the Mountains: Community-Based Coalitions for Cancer Prevention and Control* (Washington, DC: NCI, 1994).

21. Marshall et al., *Health Disparities in Appalachia;* Tompkins et al., "If You Are Old Enough"; Tina Kruger et al., "Perceptions of Smoking Cessation Programs in Rural Appalachia," *American Journal of Health Behavior* 36, no. 3 (2012): 373–84; Nancy Schoenberg et al., "Perspectives on Healthy Eating among Appalachian Residents," *Journal of Rural Health* 29, suppl. 1 (2013): s25–34; Michael Meyer, Mary Toborg, Sharon Denham, and Mary Mande, "Cultural Perspectives Concerning Adolescent Use of Tobacco and Alcohol in the Appalachian Mountain Region," *Journal of Rural Health* 24, no. 1 (2008): 67–74; Beatty et al., *Health Disparities Related to Obesity;* East Tennessee State University and NORC, *Health Disparities Related to Smoking;* J. Travis Donahoe, Andrea Titus, and Nancy Fleischer, "Key Factors Inhibiting Legislative Progress toward Smoke-Free Coverage in Appalachia," *American Journal of Public Health* 108, no. 3 (2018): 372–78.

22. East Tennessee State University and NORC, *Health Disparities Related to Smoking;* Kruger et al., "Perceptions of Smoking Cessation Programs"; Donahoe et al., "Key Factors Inhibiting Legislative Progress"; W. Jay Christian, Courtney Walker, Bin Huang, and Ellen Hahn, "Effect of Local Smoke-Free Ordinances on Smoking Prevalence in Kentucky, 2002–

2009," *Southern Medical Journal* 112, no. 7 (2019): 369–75; Ellen Hahn et al., "A Controlled Community-Based Trial to Promote Smoke-Free Policy in Rural Communities," *Journal of Rural Health* 31, no. 1 (2015): 76–88; Ellen Hahn, Mary Kay Rayens, and Nancy York, "Readiness for Smoke-Free Policy and Overall Strength of Tobacco Control in Rural Tobacco-Growing Communities," *Health Promotion Practice* 14, no. 2 (2013): 238–46; Mary Kay Rayens et al., "Political Climate and Smoke-Free Laws in Rural Kentucky Communities," *Policy, Politics & Nursing Practice* 13, no. 2 (2012): 90–97; Amanda Fallin et al., "A Short Online Community Readiness Survey for Smoke-Free Policy," *Nicotine & Tobacco Research* 14, no. 12 (2012): 1494–98; Tompkins et al., "If You Are Old Enough"; Sherry Liu et al., "Risk Perceptions of Smokeless Tobacco among Adolescent and Adult Users and Nonusers," *Journal of Health Communication* 20, no. 5 (2015): 599–606.

23. Beatty et al., *Health Disparities Related to Obesity;* Marshall et al., *Health Disparities in Appalachia;* Jaime Booth, Kai Wei, and Allison Little, "Examining the Impact of Food Environment Changes on County-Level Obesity Prevalence in the Appalachian Region," *Journal of Health Disparities Research and Practice* 10, no. 4 (2017): 14–33; Schoenberg et al., "Perspectives on Healthy Eating"; Beatty et al., *Health Disparities Related to Obesity;* Rice et al., "Beliefs about Behavioral Determinants of Obesity."

24. Vanderpool et al., "Cancer-Related Beliefs."

25. Vanderpool et al., "Fatalistic Beliefs and Completion"; Kristin Mark, Richard Crosby, and Robin Vanderpool, "Psychosocial Correlates of Ever Having a Pap Test and Abnormal Pap Results in a Sample of Rural Appalachian Women," *Journal of Rural Health* 34, no. 2 (2018): 148–54; Hutson et al., "Mountains Hold Things In."

26. Arlene Fink, *Evidence-Based Public Health Practice* (Thousand Oaks, CA: Sage Publications, 2013).

27. Rodriguez et al., "Social-Ecological Review of Cancer Disparities"; Vanderpool et al., "Adapting and Implementing Evidence-Based Cancer Education"; Behringer and Friedell, "Appalachia: Where Place Matters in Health"; Donahoe et al., "Key Factors Inhibiting Legislative Progress"; East Tennessee State University and NORC, *Health Disparities Related to Smoking;* National Association of County and City Health Officials, "Mobilizing Action through Planning and Partnership," 2012, https://www.naccho.org/programs/public-health -infrastructure/performance-improvement/community-health-assessment/mapp; Charles F. Kettering Foundation, "Naming and Framing Difficult Issues to Make Sound Decisions," 2011, https://www.kettering.org/wp-content/uploads/Naming_Framing_2011-.pdf; Lyle Wray and Paul Epstein, "Harnessing the Power of Community Collaborations," *Public Management* 94, no. 2 (2012): 94; Julie Jacobs et al., "Tools for Implementing an Evidence-Based Approach in Public Health Practice," *Preventing Chronic Disease* 9 (2012): E116; Fink, *Evidence-Based Public Health Practice.*

28. Jacobs et al., "Tools for Implementing an Evidence-Based Approach"; Felipe González Castro, Manuel Barrera, and Charles Martinez, "The Cultural Adaptation of Prevention Interventions: Resolving Tensions between Fidelity and Fit," *Prevention Science* 5, no. 1 (2004): 41–45; Beatty et al., *Health Disparities Related to Obesity;* East Tennessee State University and NORC, *Health Disparities Related to Smoking;* NCI, Cancer Control P.L.A.N.E.T., https://cancercontrolplanet.cancer.gov/planet/; Vanderpool et al., "Adapting and Implementing Evidence-Based Cancer Education"; Meyer et al., "Cultural Perspectives."

29. Nancy Schoenberg et al., "A Randomized Controlled Trial of a Faith-Placed, Lay Health Advisor Delivered Smoking Cessation Intervention for Rural Residents," *Preventive Medicine* 3 (2016): 317–23.

30. American College of Obstetricians and Gynecologists, "ACOG Committee Opinion: Smoking Cessation during Pregnancy," October 2017, https://www.acog.org/Clinical-Guidance-and-Publications/Committee-Opinions/Committee-on-Obstetric-Practice/Smoking-Cessation-During-Pregnancy; Clinical Practice Guideline Treating Tobacco Use and Dependence Update Panel, Liaisons, and Staff, "A Clinical Practice Guideline for Treating Tobacco Use and Dependence: 2008 Update. A U.S. Public Health Service Report," *American Journal of Preventive Medicine* 35, no. 2 (2008): 158–76; Ilana Chertok, Megan Casey, and Kimberly Greenfield, "Approach to Addressing Prenatal Smoking in West Virginia," *West Virginia Medical Journal* 110, no. 4 (2014): 36–40.

31. Rural Health Information Hub, "Spit It Out–West Virginia," February 27, 2017, https://www.ruralhealthinfo.org/project-examples/634.

32. CDC, "Smokefree Policies Improve Health," January 17, 2018, https://www.cdc.gov/tobacco/data_statistics/fact_sheets/secondhand_smoke/protection/improve_health/index.htm; Hahn et al., "Readiness for Smoke-Free Policy"; Christian et al., "Effect of Local Smoke-Free Ordinances."

33. Electra Paskett et al., "A Group Randomized Trial to Reduce Obesity among Appalachian Church Members: The Walk by Faith Study," *Cancer Epidemiology, Biomarkers, and Prevention* 27, no. 11 (2018): 1289–97; Nancy Schoenberg, "Enhancing the Role of Faith-Based Organizations to Improve Health: A Commentary," *Translational Behavioral Medicine* 7, no. 3 (2017): 529–31.

34. Timothy McKnight et al., "Assessing Effectiveness and Cost Benefit of the Trinity Hospital Twin City Fit for Life Program for Weight Loss and Diabetes Prevention in a Rural Midwestern Town," *Preventing Chronic Disease* 15 (2018): E98; Rural Health Information Hub, "Trinity Hospital Twin City's Fit for Life 2018," November 19, 2018, https://www.ruralhealthinfo.org/project-examples/851.

35. McKnight et al., "Assessing Effectiveness and Cost Benefit."

36. Smith and Holloman, "Piloting 'Sodabriety.'"

37. Alison Gustafson et al., "Community-Wide Efforts to Improve the Consumer Food Environment and Physical Activity Resources in Rural Kentucky," *Preventing Chronic Disease* 16 (2019): E07; Emily DeWitt et al., "A Community-Based Marketing Campaign at Farmers Markets to Encourage Fruit and Vegetable Purchases in Rural Counties with High Rates of Obesity, Kentucky, 2015–2016," *Preventing Chronic Disease* 14 (2017): E72; Emily Liu, Tammy Stephenson, Jessica Houlihan, and Alison Gustafson, "Marketing Strategies to Encourage Rural Residents of High-Obesity Counties to Buy Fruits and Vegetables in Grocery Stores," *Preventing Chronic Disease* 14 (2017): E94.

38. Michael Kanter et al., "Proactive Office Encounter: A Systematic Approach to Preventive and Chronic Care at Every Patient Encounter," *Permanente Journal* 14, no. 3 (2010): 38–43; Vanderpool et al., "Adaptation of an Evidence-Based Intervention"; Michael Kanter, Gail Lindsay, Jim Bellows, and Alide Chase, "Complete Care at Kaiser Permanente: Transforming Chronic and Preventive Care," *Joint Commission Journal on Quality and Patient Safety* 39, no. 11 (2013): 484–94.

39. Vanderpool et al., "Adaptation of an Evidence-Based Intervention"; Angela Carman, Robin Vanderpool, Lindsay Stradtman, and Emily Edmiston, "A Change-Management Approach to Closing Care Gaps in a Federally Qualified Health Center: A Rural Kentucky Case Study," *Preventing Chronic Disease* 16 (2019): E105.

40. Teresa Gardner, Paul Gavaza, Paula Meade, and Donna Adkins, "Delivering Free Healthcare to Rural Central Appalachia Population: The Case of the Health Wagon," *Rural and Remote Health* 12 (2012): 2035.

41. Health Wagon, "2018 Annual Report: Delivering Health Care to Southwest Virginia," 2019, https://zcyfq2mbiye25zfx32ieu591-wpengine.netdna-ssl.com/wp-content/uploads/2019/10/HW_2018AnnualReport_Web.pdf; Gardner et al., "Delivering Free Healthcare."

42. Rural Health Information Hub, "Kentucky Homeplace," January 28, 2015, https://www.ruralhealthinfo.org/project-examples/785; Roberto Cardarelli et al., "Terminate Lung Cancer (TLC) Study—A Mixed-Methods Population Approach to Increase Lung Cancer Screening Awareness and Low-Dose Computed Tomography in Eastern Kentucky," *Cancer Epidemiology* 46 (2017): 1–8; Frances Feltner, Sydney Thompson, William Baker, and Melissa Slone, "Community Health Workers Improving Diabetes Outcomes in a Rural Appalachian Population," *Social Work in Health Care* 56, no. 2 (2017): 115–23; Frances Feltner et al., "Effectiveness of Community Health Workers in Providing Outreach and Education for Colorectal Cancer Screening in Appalachian Kentucky," *Social Work in Health Care* 51, no. 5 (2012): 430–40.

43. Vanderpool and Huang, "Cancer Risk Perceptions"; Vanderpool et al., "Cancer-Related Beliefs"; Behringer and Friedell, "Appalachia: Where Place Matters in Health"; Schoenberg et al., "Randomized Controlled Trial"; Paskett et al., "Group Randomized Trial"; Electra Paskett et al., "Disparities in Underserved White Populations: The Case of Cancer-Related Disparities in Appalachia," *Oncologist* 16, no. 8 (2011): 1072–81; Donahoe et al., "Key Factors Inhibiting Legislative Progress"; Beatty et al., *Health Disparities Related to Obesity;* East Tennessee State University and NORC, *Health Disparities Related to Smoking.*

6

The Availability of Health Care in Appalachia

RICHARD C. INGRAM, RACHEL HOGG-GRAHAM,
TIMOTHY WILLIAMS, AND KATHERINE YOUNGEN

The Appalachian region lags behind much of the rest of the United States in many of the social and ecological determinants of health and associated health outcomes. A combination of economic, behavioral, and cultural characteristics likely contributes to these disparities. As noted earlier in the book, evidence suggests that many areas of Appalachia have made strides in the past few decades in improving the determinants of health and, as a consequence, health status (though at a slower rate than the rest of the nation). However, lack of access to health care services aggravates the health-related challenges faced by many in Appalachia and makes it harder to improve health status by both preventing and treating disease. In response, stakeholders have mounted local and national efforts to improve access to care for residents of the region. Access includes several components—financial, geographic, cultural, and convenience—all of which contribute to the health disparities that exist in Appalachia. This chapter develops these notions of access and disparities as they relate to the health of Appalachia's people.[1]

Impact of the Patient Protection and Affordable Care Act in Appalachia

The Patient Protection and Affordable Care Act (ACA) sought to improve access to health care in the United States by expanding the number of Americans covered by health insurance and by increasing the health care workforce.

Medicaid Expansion

One pillar of the ACA was the expansion of Medicaid eligibility to nonelderly adults with incomes up to 138 percent of the federal poverty level. Evidence suggests that, even prior to enactment of the ACA, many parts of Appalachia had relatively favorable insurance rates when compared with the rest of the nation. However, there were also areas with distressingly low rates of coverage, where less than 60 percent of the nonelderly population had insurance. These areas were located mostly in the West Virginia counties in the North Central region of Appalachia, the North Carolina counties in the South Central region, and the South Carolina, Georgia, and Mississippi counties that make up much of the Southern region. Given the significant disparities in access to health care between Appalachia and the rest of the nation, Medicaid expansion presented an opportunity to radically increase the availability of health care services to Appalachia's residents. However, many of the states in Appalachia with the greatest need failed to embrace Medicaid expansion as a mechanism to increase access to health care.[2]

Of the thirteen states that have counties located in the Appalachian region, seven initially declined to expand Medicaid (Virginia eventually moved to do so in 2018). All the states that declined to expand Medicaid were located in the South and South Central subregions of Appalachia. This failure to expand Medicaid was a missed opportunity to increase access to health care services in an area with a particularly high need. In Appalachia, nonexpansion states had higher rates of uninsured nonelderly residents than expansion states before the ACA was implemented (19 percent versus 15 percent in 2010), suggesting that expansion could have had a particularly large impact in these areas. The national rate of uninsured among the nonelderly population was 18 percent in 2010.[3]

Medicaid expansion substantially reduced the uninsured rates in expansion states in Appalachia in comparison to their nonexpansion counterparts. Estimates suggest that the national rate of uninsured nonelderly people decreased 38 percent from 2010 to 2015. The uninsured rate in nonexpansion states dropped approximately 30 percent between 2010 and 2015 (due in part to the increased availability of health insurance through state-based exchanges funded through the ACA), while the uninsured rate in expansion states dropped approximately 42 percent. This disparity had serious implications for many Americans—the average number of uninsured nonelderly adults in nonexpansion states dropped by 315,000, while the average drop in expansion states was 482,000. Given the historically high rate of uninsured individuals in Appalachian counties, the expansion of Medicaid could have been a particularly effective means of increasing access to health care, yet policy decisions left many in the region unable to take advantage.[4]

Although many states that contain Appalachian counties fared relatively poorly compared with the rest of the nation in terms of health insurance coverage, the Appalachian region as a whole fared relatively well. Table 6.1 displays the percentage of adults without health insurance in Appalachian and non-Appalachian counties in 2010, before the expansion of Medicaid, and in 2016, two years after the ACA was fully implemented. Prior to expansion, the

Table 6.1. Percentage of Adults without Health Insurance before (2010) and after (2016) the ACA

	Appalachian Counties	Non-Appalachian Counties	Difference	% Difference
2010	22.18	22.35	−0.16	0.74
2016	12.18	13.46	−1.28	10.491
% Difference	45.09	39.77		
Females Aged 18–64 Uninsured				
2010	20.30	20.38	−0.09	0.42
2016	10.51	11.87	−1.36	12.96
% Difference	48.22	41.76		
Males Aged 18–64 Uninsured				
2010	24.10	24.33	−0.23	0.949
2016	13.88	15.06	−1.18	8.486
% Difference	42.42	38.12		

overall percentage of uninsured adults in Appalachia was slightly lower in all demographic categories examined (all adults, adult females, and adult males). However, the difference between Appalachian and non-Appalachian counties was minimal: less than 1 percent in all categories examined.

Although Appalachian counties had a slight pre-ACA advantage in the percentage of the adult population uninsured, they were able to reduce the proportion of uninsured to a greater extent than their non-Appalachian counterparts. Between 2010 and 2016, Appalachian counties saw a 45.09 percent reduction in uninsured adults (from 22.18 to 12.18 percent). The reduction in the rest of the United States was substantial but of a smaller magnitude: 39.77 percent (from 22.35 to 13.46 percent).

The reduction in uninsured adults from 2010 to 2016 disproportionately benefited women—even though a higher percentage of women than men were insured. In 2010, 20.30 and 20.38 percent of Appalachian and non-Appalachian women, respectively, were uninsured. In contrast, 24.10 and 24.33 percent of Appalachian and non-Appalachian men, respectively, were uninsured. In 2016 the percentage of uninsured women in Appalachian counties had almost been cut in half, to 10.51 percent; the percentage of uninsured women in non-Appalachian counties dropped to 11.87 percent, a reduction of 41.76 percent. The reduction among males was more modest. In 2016 the percentage of uninsured men in Appalachian counties dropped by 42.42 percent, to 13.88 percent; the percentage of uninsured men in non-Appalachian counties dropped to 15.06 percent, a reduction of 38.12 percent.

Provider Availability

To meet the projected increased need for providers resulting from better access to health care driven by higher numbers of insured, the ACA included provisions to increase the number of health care workers in the United States. These provisions included initiatives to support the training of health care, dental, and behavioral health providers and to incentivize them to practice in medically underserved areas upon graduation. These provisions had the potential to substantially increase the number of providers in the Appalachian region.[5]

Table 6.2 displays the mean number of professionals in selected occupations in Appalachian and non-Appalachian counties in the United States before and after implementation of the ACA. Prior to its enactment, non-Appalachian counties averaged higher numbers of providers in all categories examined. The difference in mean number of providers per county ranged from 48.5 to 164 percent.

Table 6.3 displays changes in the mean number of professionals before and after the ACA in Appalachian and non-Appalachian counties. Both Appalachian and non-Appalachian counties saw an increase in provider numbers for all categories examined—ranging from 0.97 to 105.14 percent in Appalachian counties and from 4.28 to 86.57 percent in non-Appalachian counties. Both Appalachian and non-Appalachian counties saw a particularly large increase in physician assistants (PAs), advance practice registered nurses (APRNs), and nurse practitioners (NPs). It is important to note that APRNs encompass four specialties: nurse practitioners, clinical nurse specialists, nurse midwives, and nurse anesthetists. These increases may have been due in part to provisions of the ACA that specifically targeted these professions and provided funding for care delivery models that used these types of providers, such as nurse-managed health clinics.[6]

One reason for the lower number of providers in Appalachian counties might be due to population—many Appalachian counties are sparsely populated. Table 6.4 displays the mean number of selected health care professionals per 10,000 population in Appalachian and non-Appalachian counties. When population is taken into account, Appalachian counties compare more favorably to the rest of the nation; however, in general, Appalachian counties still lag behind non-Appalachian counties. The difference in mean number of providers per 10,000 population between Appalachian and non-Appalachian counties in 2010, before the ACA was enacted, ranged from 7.14 to 15.33 percent for the professions examined. However, the mean number of APRNs and NPs per 10,000 population was 15.33 and 12.46 percent higher in Appalachia, respectively.

Table 6.2. Mean Number of Selected Health Care Professionals per County in Appalachian and Non-Appalachian Counties, 2010 versus 2016

	2010			2016		
Occupation	Appalachian	Non-Appalachian	% Difference	Appalachian	Non-Appalachian	% Difference
PCP	38.79	75.89	95.64	40.51	82.04	102.72
PA	14.09	24.46	73.53	22.56	38.38	70.12
APRN	33.99	50.48	48.51	59.29	86.35	45.64
NP	21.03	36.10	71.66	43.14	67.35	56.12
Dentist	26.26	61.52	134.23	30.00	73.74	145.80
OB-GYN	5.16	12.38	139.92	5.21	12.91	147.79
PED	6.90	18.26	164.64	7.24	19.38	167.68
CNM	0.73	1.72	135.62	0.85	2.34	175.29

Table 6.3. Mean Number of Selected Health Care Professionals per County in 2010 and 2016, Appalachian versus Non-Appalachian Counties

	Appalachian			Non-Appalachian		
Occupation	2010	2016	% Difference	2010	2016	% Difference
PCP	38.79	40.51	4.43	75.89	82.04	8.10
PA	14.09	22.56	60.11	24.46	38.38	56.91
APRN	33.99	59.29	74.43	50.48	86.35	71.06
NP	21.03	43.14	105.14	36.10	67.35	86.57
Dentist	26.26	30.00	14.24	61.52	73.74	19.86
OB-GYN	5.16	5.21	0.97	12.38	12.91	4.28
PED	6.90	7.24	4.93	18.26	19.38	6.13
CNM	0.73	0.85	16.44	1.72	2.34	36.05

Table 6.5 displays changes in the mean number of professionals per 10,000 population before and after the ACA in Appalachian and non-Appalachian counties. Between 2010 and 2016, Appalachian counties experienced higher rates of growth per 10,000 population in three of the eight professions examined.

Of particular note are the disparities in the availability of professionals who provide primary care, including primary care physicians (PCPs), PAs, and NPs. In 2010 the mean number of PCPs (excluding pediatricians) per 10,000 population in non-Appalachian counties was 7.39 percent higher than in Appalachian counties, and the mean number of pediatricians (PEDs) per

Table 6.4. Mean Number of Selected Health Care Professionals per 10,000 Residents in Appalachian and Non-Appalachian Counties, 2010 versus 2016

	2010			2016		
Occupation	Appalachian	Non-Appalachian	% Difference	Appalachian	Non-Appalachian	% Difference
PCP	5.01	5.38	7.39	4.89	5.31	8.59
PA	1.82	1.95	7.14	2.74	2.66	2.92
APRN	4.37	3.70	15.33	7.54	5.99	20.56
NP	3.13	2.74	12.46	6.06	4.82	20.46
Dentist	3.18	3.79	19.18	3.58	4.41	23.18
OB-GYN	0.48	0.53	10.42	0.46	0.51	10.87
PED	0.64	0.71	10.94	0.64	0.71	10.94
CNM	0.09	0.10	11.11	0.11	0.12	9.09

Table 6.5. Mean Number of Selected Health Care Professionals per 10,000 Residents in 2010 and 2016, Appalachian versus Non-Appalachian Counties

	Appalachian			Non-Appalachian		
Occupation	2010	2016	% Difference	2010	2016	% Difference
PCP	5.01	4.89	2.4	5.38	5.31	1.30
PA	1.82	2.74	50.55	1.95	2.66	36.41
APRN	4.37	7.54	72.54	3.70	5.99	61.89
NP	3.13	6.06	93.61	2.74	4.82	75.91
Dentist	3.18	3.58	12.58	3.79	4.41	16.36
OB-GYN	0.48	0.46	−4.17	0.53	0.51	−3.77
PED	0.64	0.64	0.00	0.71	0.71	0.00
CNM	0.09	0.11	22.22	0.10	0.12	20.00

10,000 population was 10.94 percent higher. The mean number of PAs was 7.14 percent higher in non-Appalachian than in Appalachian counties. However, the mean number of NPs per 10,000 population was 12.46 percent higher in Appalachian counties.

Both Appalachian and non-Appalachian counties saw a noticeable growth in the mean number of PAs and NPs per 10,000 population between 2010 and 2016; however, Appalachian counties saw higher rates of growth in three professions. The change in the mean number of PAs per 10,000 population in Appalachian counties during that period was substantial—50.55 percent—compared with 36.41 percent in non-Appalachian counties. The change in mean number of NPs per 10,000 population was noticeably higher in Appalachian counties (93.61 percent) than in non-Appalachian counties (75.91 percent). In contrast, the mean number of PCPs per 10,000 population fell in both regions, and the mean number of PEDs stayed stable in both regions.

Despite the notable increase in the number of health care providers in Appalachia from 2010 to 2016, disparities remain in the mean number of primary care providers per 10,000 population. Gaps between Appalachian and non-Appalachian counties grew for PCPs and NPs. In 2016 the mean number of PCPs per 10,000 population was 8.59 percent higher in non-Appalachian counties than in Appalachian counties, and the mean number of NPs per 10,000 population was 20.46 percent higher. However, Appalachian counties were able to close the gap in mean number of PAs per 10,000 population, which fell to 2.92 percent. The mean number of PEDs per 10,000 population stayed the same, at 10.94 percent.

There are also disparities in the availability of professionals who can provide obstetric and gynecologic care, including obstetrician-gynecologists (OB-GYNs) and certified nurse midwives (CNMs), between Appalachian and non-Appalachian counties. These disparities are particularly concerning given the inequities in birth outcomes and the high rates of cervical cancer seen in the Appalachian region. Table 6.2 shows that in 2010 the mean number of OB-GYNs and CNMs in non-Appalachian counties was more than 130 percent higher than in Appalachian counties. Even after accounting for population, non-Appalachian counties still have significant advantages over their Appalachian peers—in 2010 the mean number of OB-GYNs and CNMs were 10.42 percent and 11.11 percent higher in non-Appalachian counties, respectively.[7]

Both Appalachian and non-Appalachian counties saw decreases in OB-GYNs and increases in CNMs per 10,000 population between 2010 and 2016. However, the mean number of OB-GYNs per 10,000 population declined at a lower rate in non-Appalachian counties than in Appalachian counties (3.77 versus 4.17 percent). In contrast, the mean number of CNMs per 10,000 population in Appalachian counties grew at a faster rate than in non-Appalachian counties (22.22 versus 20.00 percent).

Given the modest increases in the number of OB-GYNs and CNMs in the Appalachian region, it should come as no surprise that disparities between Appalachian and non-Appalachian counties remain. In 2016 the mean number of OB-GYNs per 10,000 population in non-Appalachian counties was 10.87 percent higher than in Appalachian counties. The mean number of CNMs per 10,000 population in non-Appalachian counties was 9.09 percent higher than in Appalachian counties.

The availability of dentists in the Appalachian region also lags behind the rest of the nation. This is particularly concerning, given that Appalachia has poorer oral health outcomes than much of the United States. Unmet dental needs are serious, often resulting in chronic pain, emergency department visits, and prescriptions for pain medications—contributing to the opioid misuse discussed in chapter 9. Table 6.4 shows that prior to enactment of the ACA, the mean number of dentists per 10,000 population in non-Appalachian counties was almost 20 percent higher than in Appalachian counties. Table 6.5 shows that between 2010 and 2016 the percentage of growth in the mean number of dentists per 10,000 population in Appalachian and non-Appalachian counties was substantial (12.58 and 16.36 percent, respectively). Regional disparities widened slightly after passage of the ACA, with the mean number of dentists per 10,000 population in non-Appalachian counties a little more than 23 percent higher than in Appalachian counties. In the case of dentists, higher numbers do not automatically translate to better access, as many dentists in Appalachia do not participate in Medicaid. Moreover, dental reimbursement rates did not change appreciably in Appalachia after implementation of the ACA.[8]

Restrictions on the Scope of Practice of Nonphysician and Nondentist Providers

Evidence suggests that nonphysician providers such as NPs, PAs, and CNMs often deliver care that is indistinguishable from that provided by physicians, and it may be more accessible to those living in rural areas. Given the relative lack of availability of primary care physicians, Appalachian states might be expected to explore ways to increase the delivery of health care by nonphysician and nondentist providers such as NPs, PAs, and dental therapists. However, this does not appear to be the case.[9]

Many Appalachian states have tight restrictions on the scope of practice for these types of providers. Twelve of the thirteen states in Appalachia restrict NPs' scope of practice to a greater extent than that recommended by the National Academy of Medicine; they restrict the activities of NPs in areas such as independent practice, diagnostic testing, and prescribing. Similar issues exist for PAs. Eleven of the thirteen states in Appalachia have restrictions in three or more areas related to prescribing authority, scope of practice, co-signing by physicians, and supervision of PAs. CNMs face challenges related to scope of practice as well. Ten of thirteen Appalachian states give CNMs less autonomy than their peers in much of the rest of the United States.[10]

The restrictive practice environments of NPs, PAs, and CNMs in Appalachia have serious implications for patient access. The number of students choosing careers in these areas is growing, and it is much higher than the number of medical school graduates choosing primary care residencies. Many see these nonphysician professionals as critical to increasing the health care workforce and improving access to health care services. However, evidence suggests that these nonphysician providers are less likely to locate in areas where their scope of practice is restricted and they have less autonomy. Thus, many Appalachian states have created an environment that discourages nonphysician providers from practicing in them.[11]

Given disparities in the availability of dentists, Appalachian states might be expected to embrace more liberal scope-of-practice models that do not limit the provision of dental care to dentists. Dental hygienists, for instance, are licensed and trained oral health care professionals who can provide services such as cleaning and examination. However, many Appalachian states lag behind the rest of the nation when it comes to expanding the scope of practice for hygienists; nine of the thirteen Appalachian states have scope-of-practice regulations for hygienists that are less favorable than those in much of the rest of the United States. Appalachian states have also failed to embrace other models that can expand access to basic dental care, such as the use of dental therapists.[12]

Hospital Availability

Poor access to care related to provider availability may be compounded by a relative lack of hospitals in Appalachia. In 2016, the most recent year for which data were available, the mean number of hospitals per 10,000 population in Appalachia was 0.31, or just over half the rate in the rest of the country (0.54 per 10,000). Limited access to hospitals in Appalachia can have serious impacts on the health of residents. Evidence suggests that longer travel times to hospitals are associated with poor health outcomes and decreased access to health care services.[13]

Rural hospital closures are becoming increasingly common throughout the United States: 160 rural hospitals closed from 2005 to 2019. Evidence suggests that these closures carry significant implications for patient health, and they disproportionately impact rural areas. Rural hospital closures are associated with increased travel time to hospitals, which can result in poor birth outcomes, difficulty obtaining trauma care, and poor cardiovascular health outcomes. One analysis found that, after the closure of a rural hospital, it took patients in that zip code an average of eleven minutes more to get to a hospital in an ambulance following a 911 call. In contrast, residents of urban and suburban areas saw no increase in travel times. Hospital closures in rural areas are

Table 6.6. Hospital Closures in Appalachia, 2005–2019

State	Closures in Appalachian Counties	Total Closures
Alabama*	3	7
Georgia*	2	8
Kentucky	3	5
Maryland	0	0
Mississippi*	1	6
New York	2	5
North Carolina*	5	11
Ohio	1	2
Pennsylvania	4	4
South Carolina*	0	4
Tennessee*	8	13
Virginia*	2	2
West Virginia	3	3

*Non–Medicaid expansion states in 2014.

also associated with a substantial decrease in the supply of physicians, particularly primary care physicians.[14]

The loss of a hospital can dramatically affect not only access to health care but also the economic health of a community. Hospitals are significant drivers of economic activity in many rural areas, and their closures can add to health and economic inequities in the area. Evidence suggests that hospital closures can lead to both decreased per capita income and increased unemployment rates. This could worsen the already significant health disparities present in many rural communities.[15]

Table 6.6 displays the number of hospital closures in Appalachian counties from 2005 to 2019. Of the 160 rural hospital closures reported since 2005, 70 have been in the states that make up the Appalachian region, and 34 have occurred in Appalachian counties. Tennessee and North Carolina experienced the highest number of closures in Appalachian counties (eight and five, respectively). This may be due, in part, to the lack of Medicaid expansion in these states. Nine of the twenty-one hospital closures in Appalachian counties in nonexpansion states occurred after 2015—the rest occurred before Medicaid expansion was enacted in 2014. In contrast, only three of the thirteen hospital closures in Appalachian counties in Medicaid expansion states occurred after those states implemented Medicaid expansion. Evidence suggests that a state's decision to expand Medicaid is associated with less uncompensated care, which may help improve a hospital's financial viability, and it is associated with a lower likelihood of rural hospital closures. Failing to expand Medicaid eligibility may have been a lost opportunity for states to prevent rural hospital closures.[16]

The disparity is even more pronounced between Appalachia and the rest of the United States in the case of critical access hospitals (CAHs). Congress created the CAH designation under the Balanced Budget Act of 1997 in reaction to a rash of rural hospital closures in the 1980s and 1990s. CAHs are rural hospitals that must generally be located more than thirty-five miles from other hospitals, provide twenty-four-hour emergency care, have no more than twenty-five acute care inpatient beds, and, with some exceptions, provide inpatient care for no longer than ninety-six hours on average. Hospitals with the CAH designation are eligible to receive from Medicare 101 percent of allowable costs—a reimbursement system that differs markedly from the standard rates based on the type and number of services provided. This reimbursement system was intended to improve the financial viability of CAHs by decreasing the financial risk associated with payment based on fixed rates for specific procedures and specific conditions.[17]

Given the low levels of access to health care services and relative lack of economic resources in much of Appalachia, it might be reasonable to expect hospitals in the region to embrace CAH designation as a means of preserving access to care by reducing financial instability. Available data indicate that this is not the case. In 2016, the latest year for which data were available, Appalachian counties had 0.12 CAHs per 10,000 residents; the rate in non-Appalachian counties was 242 percent higher, at 0.42 per 10,000. Of the thirty-four rural hospitals that closed in Appalachia between 2005 and 2019, fifteen were CAHs. The Appalachian region clearly lags behind the rest of the nation in the presence of CAHs, suggesting that this is an underutilized mechanism for preserving hospitals' financial viability.

Improving Access to Health Care Services

The lack of access to health care services in Appalachia today is a continuation of long-standing issues. Disparities in the social and ecological determinants of health—particularly poverty, geography, and behavior—create a negative feedback loop that results in and exacerbates disparities between rural and urban areas. This has been the case in Appalachia since the early days of European settlement, and many efforts have been undertaken to improve health in the region.[18]

Frontier Nursing Service

The idea for the Frontier Nursing Service (FNS) sprang from the experiences of its founder, Mary Breckinridge, shortly after the end of World War I. She was a trained nurse and had served as a public health nurse in Washington, DC. Breckinridge later traveled to France with the American Committee for Devastated France and engaged in a number of public health and maternal and child health initiatives, including disaster relief and activities focused on children and pregnant women. While in France, she also founded a public health nursing service and was exposed to the British practice of combining nursing and midwifery.[19]

Upon returning to the United States, Breckinridge continued her education by taking classes in public health and nursing at Columbia University's Teachers College. Thinking that the integrated nursing-midwifery model she had seen in Europe would be an effective way to improve health outcomes in rural America, she returned to England to study midwifery, and she received certification as a midwife in 1924. While in England, she traveled to Scotland to observe the workings of a nurse-centric health care organization that served the largely rural Scottish Highlands and Inner and Outer Hebrides. Between taking courses at Columbia and studying midwifery in England, Breckinridge traveled through the mountains of eastern Kentucky to observe the "granny midwives" practicing in the region. She observed that although these practitioners lacked formal training and used empirical methods and folk medicine, they actively managed the labor of their patients and intervened when the women experienced complications during or after birth. She also concluded that, given the lack of physicians in many rural parts of eastern Kentucky, it would be an ideal place to demonstrate the effectiveness of using trained midwives not only to deliver babies but also to provide basic prenatal, postnatal, and pediatric health care services.

Once she returned from England, Breckinridge established the Kentucky Committee for Mothers and Babies (which later became the FNS) in Leslie County, Kentucky. Leslie County was a particularly needy place. It had no health care infrastructure (there were no licensed physicians) and lacked railroad access and electricity. The area was also extremely poor—the average annual income was less than 25 percent of the Southern Appalachian average and less than 15 percent of the national average. Breckinridge's original vison was for a much more expansive project that would serve a much larger part of the region. However, due to resistance from some in the medical community (in particular, the head of the Kentucky Bureau of Child and Maternal Health), the committee was unable to obtain money from the Commonwealth Fund and instead had to cobble together a network of small private donors. In spite of these setbacks, the FNS opened a clinic in Hyden, Kentucky, in 1925 (which later became Mary Breckinridge Hospital and was eventually sold to Appalachian Regional Health). The FNS clinic model was based on the structure used by the American Committee for Devastated France to deliver health care services. The FNS model also relied heavily on community engagement; community advisory committees were established to meet local residents, gain trust and support in the communities served by the FNS, and deliver culturally competent care that respected the mountain culture. By 1965, the FNS infrastructure had grown to a twenty-seven-bed hospital and five satellite nursing centers.

The FNS had an almost immediate impact on the health of Leslie County and surrounding areas. Maternal death was a major cause of death in the region prior to the founding of the FNS, but there were no maternal deaths in the first 1,000 deliveries performed by FNS staff. The maternal mortality rate associated with FNS deliveries from its founding to 1934 was 0.68 per 1,000 live births; the national maternal mortality rate during that time was between 5.6 and 6.8 per 1,000 live births. The rate of prenatal and postnatal complications was lower than the national average, and the rates of maternal and neonatal deaths and stillbirths from 1950 to 1970 were lower for FNS patients than in Kentucky overall. These numbers are particularly impressive because many of the mothers seen by the FNS were considered high-risk patients. The area served by the FNS eventually grew to encompass almost 700 square miles.[20]

In addition, the FNS provided preventive care to the patients it served, including inoculations for diseases such as typhoid, tetanus, and diphtheria. It also supplied health education on a diverse array of topics, including nutrition and sanitation. It is important to note that the FNS provided these services not just for mothers and babies but for the entire family.[21]

The rapid growth and success of the FNS suggest that its model of nurse-centric care was both viable and effective. However, the FNS was unable to obtain sufficient financial backing to expand operations. In addition to resistance from the medical community, it fell victim to larger world events. The Great Depression damaged the Southern Appalachian subregion's already struggling economy. Many people were unable to afford food, and the Depression made it harder to obtain funds from donors to help the needy. Food insecurity in the region was aggravated by a severe drought that made it hard to grow subsistence crops. In spite of decreased funds and increased demand, the FNS remained committed to helping families in need and began to operate at a large deficit. The financial difficulties resulting from the Great Depression forced the FNS to cut salaries and reduce staff. It also shelved plans to expand into the Ozarks in Arkansas and Missouri. Its ranks were further depleted when many of the nurses imported from Great Britain returned home to serve during World War II. Staffing issues continued to plague the FNS and hampered plans to expand its service area well into the 1960s.[22]

The pressures of the Great Depression and World War II placed a great strain on the FNS; however, they also drove the creation of a school of mid-wifery, which still exists today. The FNS opened a graduate school of midwifery at the hospital in Hyden in 1939. The first class was quite small—only two students enrolled in 1939— but there was clearly a demand for midwife educa-tion. The school grew quickly, enrolling an average of twelve students each year from 1940 to 1975. The Frontier Nursing University (FNU) now offers an array of degrees, including a master of science in nursing and a doctorate of nursing practice with a variety of specialties, including nurse-midwife, family nurse practitioner, women's health care nurse practitioner, and psychiatric mental health nurse practitioner. FNU also has a distance-learning format, and it has enrolled students from all fifty states, Guam, and the US Virgin Islands. To date, more than 4,000 students have graduated from FNU, and they compare favorably with graduates elsewhere in the nation. FNU graduates' pass rates for national board examinations from 2014 to 2018 were higher than those of their peers nationally.[23]

United Mine Workers of America

The FNS was unable to expand its service delivery much beyond Leslie County and surrounding areas, so other organizations stepped in to expand access to care in Appalachian Kentucky and West Virginia. Mining was a major employer in the area, and mining companies built much of the infrastructure in the region, including whole towns (see chapter 7 for more details). Although these company towns had stores and schools, health care infrastructure was lacking. Few towns had health care facilities, and the facilities that existed often lacked professional staff and equipment.

The lack of quality health care was a major point of friction between coal miners and coal companies. After the federal seizure of coal mines in response to a strike in 1946, the Truman administration sought to engage the United Mine Workers of America (UMWA) by creating the Welfare and Retirement Fund (WRF). The WRF was conceptualized in the Krug-Lewis agreement of 1946. It was funded by coal companies, which paid a royalty of five cents per ton of coal mined (doubled a year later to ten cents per ton and eventually reaching forty cents per ton by 1952). This money funded a host of health and welfare services, including rehabilitation for injured miners, temporary dis-ability payments for disabled miners and their families, medical care, and death and disaster benefits.[24]

Although the WRF's financial benefits addressed many of the economic concerns of miners and their families, they did not provide greater access to health care services. In response, the UMWA created the Miners Memorial

Hospital Association (MMHA) and built seven hospitals in eastern Kentucky, two hospitals in West Virginia, and one in Wise, Virginia. These hospitals contained more than 1,000 beds, attracted high-quality providers (by offering high salaries), and hosted residency and training programs. The new hospitals were filled with patients; however, many of them were indigent and could afford to pay little, if anything, for the services provided. High utilization by indigent populations quickly strained the MMHA budget. The financial situation was further threatened by a downturn in coal production and a flood that extensively damaged one of the MMHA facilities. In response to the MMHA's plans to close four hospitals to cut costs, Samuel McMaster Kerr, a Presbyterian minister, explored ways to keep the hospitals open. As a result of Kerr's efforts, the Presbyterian Church purchased the MMHA hospitals in 1963, primarily with federal funds from the US Area Redevelopment Administration. The MMHA hospitals were renamed Appalachian Regional Hospitals Inc. (ARH), and they preserved many of the MMHA's tenets, including a commitment to provide care to all, regardless of ability to pay.

In spite of the infusion of federal funds, ARH continued to struggle financially. State funds from Kentucky, along with funds from the federal government, were used to keep the struggling health care system afloat. These efforts paid off, and ARH enjoyed its first year of profitability in 1969. Although ARH struggled financially for much of its early existence, there is no doubt that it met its goal of providing health care to the communities it served. It recorded more than 1.2 million inpatient visits and 18.8 million outpatient visits from 1963 to 1994. ARH (renamed Appalachian Regional Healthcare in 1987) has expanded to become an integrated health care delivery system, and it now includes primary care clinics, psychiatric facilities, home health agencies, home medical equipment stores, and pharmacies.[25]

Appalachian Regional Commission

In spite of efforts by Mary Breckinridge and the UMWA to expand access to health care services, rural Kentuckians continued to suffer from poor health and a lack of economic opportunity. During a 1964 visit to Martin County, Kentucky, President Lyndon Johnson declared, "I have called for a national war on poverty. Our objective: total victory." Perhaps it is not surprising that Johnson chose to invest heavily in the region by championing and signing into law the Appalachian Regional Development Act of 1965 (ARDA). The ARDA established the Appalachian Regional Commission (ARC), which replaced John F. Kennedy's President's Appalachian Regional Commission (PARC). One of the ARC's main purposes was and is to develop the economy of the region. ARDA also emphasized building economic and social infrastructure in Appalachia.[26]

Many elements of ARDA closely mirrored recommendations made by PARC in *Appalachia: A Report by the President's Commission on Appalachia.* That report linked poor health status to economic challenges, and one of its recommendations was to develop community health centers (CHCs) to provide access to a wide range of health care services, including maternal and child health, mental health, dental, and primary care services. PARC's emphasis on regional implementation of the CHC model was part of a larger push by the Johnson administration to use CHCs to fight the War on Poverty. For instance, the Economic Opportunity Act of 1964 focused on community development. CHCs were conceptualized to address, on a national scale, the economic challenges posed by poor health. From 1965 to 1980, CHCs spread rapidly throughout the United States and were particularly concentrated in the Central Appalachian subregion.[27]

ARDA contained specific language that allowed the development of CHCs as demonstration health projects (DHPs). The act divided funding for DHPs into three categories:

1. Planning grants, used to fund planning activities necessary to develop DHPs.
2. Construction and equipment grants, used to build (or purchase) the facilities and equipment necessary to provide health care.
3. Operation grants, used to support the costs of operating a DHP (and meant to serve as a cost-sharing mechanism). These grants covered 50 percent of operational costs and, in the case of counties deemed at risk or distressed, might cover up to 70 percent or 80 percent of costs, respectively.[28]

It is difficult to find data on the total amount ARC has spent to improve health care infrastructure and access since its inception. However, evidence suggests that it invests heavily in health-related projects in the region. According to one estimate, ARC's total health-specific spending was $30.9 million on 202 projects from 2004 to 2010. Although this amount is substantial, estimates also suggest that, in keeping with PARC's original recommendations, ARC funds are used to leverage cost-sharing arrangements with other stakeholders. ARC seems to be particularly effective at motivating stakeholders to contribute. Its $30.9 million investment resulted in approximately $92 million of matching funds; more than half the projects received matching contributions of at least 50 percent of total costs. The vast majority of these funds (approximately $78 billion) came from community sources.[29]

ARC funds are used to support three primary activities: construction of new facilities and renovation of existing facilities, purchase of equipment, and operational services. More than half of ARC's health projects funded between 2004 and 2010 were operational in nature. (However, the *average* amount ARC contributed to construction and equipment activities was considerably higher than the amount spent on operational activities.) The vast majority of construction- and equipment-related projects focused on increasing access to care or improving service delivery.

In spite of ARC's emphasis on developing the infrastructure necessary to improve outcomes in Appalachia, access remains a challenge. Evidence suggests that there are still significant gaps between Appalachia and the rest of the nation in terms of availability of health care–related resources, health insurance coverage, and health care costs. These gaps are associated with poor economic and health outcomes in Appalachia. In 2004, forty years after President Johnson declared his War on Poverty, more than two-thirds of Appalachian counties in one study had health professional shortages in all or part of the county, and almost one-fifth lacked a hospital. There are also access-related disparities *within* the region, with residents in close proximity to metropolitan areas having better access to hospitals and to services such as cardiac catherization and cardiac rehabilitation. The per capita supply of PCPs, mental health providers, specialist physicians, and dentists in Appalachia is lower than in the rest of the United States, and the uninsured rate in certain areas of Appalachia is higher than in the rest of the nation. Although progress has been made, much remains to be done to close these gaps.[30]

Crafting a Solution

Appalachia compares quite favorably with the rest of the nation in terms of insurance coverage, yet significant deficits remain in health status and provider availability. These deficits likely limit the potential impact of expansive insurance coverage. However, it is possible to attract trained medical professionals to Appalachia and retain them. Evidence suggests that medical students who come from rural areas are more likely to practice in rural areas. Other students may be more likely to practice in rural areas if they are exposed to them during medical school or residency training. Increasing the number of students from Appalachia who participate in training programs for health care professions may increase the number of providers in the region.

Often, graduates of medical school, dental school, and other health care training programs are saddled with significant debt. One strategy to recruit these graduates to rural areas like Appalachia is debt relief. Evidence suggests that the high cost of medical school may incentivize physicians to practice in rural areas in exchange for financial support.[31] Programs at the federal and state levels use debt relief to entice physicians, dentists, and other providers to serve in rural areas. The National Health Service Corps (NHSC), for example, uses scholarships and loan repayment programs to entice students to practice in underserved areas, many of which are rural. The NHSC scholarship program pays students' tuition, fees, and living expenses in exchange for a two- to four-year commitment. The NHSC loan repayment program pays $60,000 in exchange for two years of service; these agreements can be renewed for a total of five years of service in exchange for a maximum of $170,000. The State Loan Repayment Program (SLRP) is a state-federal partnership that serves a similar purpose as the NHSC program. Graduates must practice in underserved areas for at least two years to receive funding. All but three states with Appalachian counties participate in the SLRP. Given the serious deficits in provider availability in Appalachia, it may make sense for Appalachian states to increase the funds available to students in exchange for their commitment to practice in the region.[32]

The Appalachian region of the United States has traditionally suffered from a lack of access to health care resources. Mary Breckinridge, the UMWA, and other leaders have taken bold and innovative steps to bring health care resources to Appalachia. However, the region still desperately needs more health care providers. The ACA opened the door for a multitude of those previously denied health insurance coverage; it is now time to continue the legacy of the FNS and UMWA and deploy innovative strategies to attract providers to the region and give the newly insured access to high-quality care.

Notes

1. Julie L. Marshall et al., *Health Disparities in Appalachia* (Washington, DC: Appalachian Regional Commission, 2017), https://www.arc.gov/assets/research_reports/Health _Disparities_in_Appalachia_August_2017.pdf; Cathy A. Coyne, Cristina Demian-Popescu, and Dana Friend, "Social and Cultural Factors Influencing Health in Southern West Virginia: A Qualitative Study," *Preventing Chronic Disease* 3, no. 4 (2006): A124; Joel A. Halverson, *Underlying Socioeconomic Factors Influencing Health Disparities in the Appalachian Region* (Washington, DC: Appalachian Regional Commission, 2008); Joel A. Halverson, Lin Ma, and E. James Hamer, *An Analysis of Disparities in Health Status and Access to Health Care in the Appalachian Region* (Washington, DC: Appalachian Regional Commission, 2004), https://www.arc.gov/research/researchreportdetails.asp?REPORT_ID=82.

2. John E. McDonough, "Health System Reform in the United States," *International Journal of Health Policy and Management* 2, no. 1 (2014): 5–8; Wolters Kluwer Editorial Staff, *The Affordable Care Act: Law, Regulatory Explanation and Analysis* (Chicago: Wolters Kluwer, 2013); PDA Inc. and the Cecil B. Sheps Center for Health Services Research, *Health Care Costs and Access Disparities in Appalachia* (Washington, DC: Appalachian Regional

Commission,   2012),   https://www.arc.gov/research/researchreportdetails.asp?REPORT
_ID=101.

3. Bowen Garrett and Anuj Gangopadhyaya, *Who Gained Health Insurance under the ACA, and Where Do They Live?* (Washington, DC: Urban Institute, 2016), https://www
.urban.org/sites/default/files/publication/86761/2001041-who-gained-health-insurance
-coverage-under-the-aca-and-where-do-they-live.pdf.

4. Garrett and Gangopadhyaya, *Who Gained Health Insurance.*

5. Taryn Morrisey, *Issue Brief: The Affordable Care Act's Public Health Workforce Provisions: Opportunities and Challenges* (Washington, DC: American Public Health Association, 2011).

6. J. Margo Brooks Carthon, Hilary Barnes, and Danielle Altares Sarik, "Federal Policies Influence Access to Primary Care and Nurse Practitioner Workforce," *Journal for Nurse Practitioners* 11, no. 5 (2015): 526–30; Darrell G. Kirch, Mackenzie K. Henderson, and Michael J. Dill, "Physician Workforce Projections in an Era of Health Care Reform," *Annual Review of Medicine* 63 (2012): 435–45; Peter D. Jacobson and Shelley A. Jazowski, "Physicians, the Affordable Care Act, and Primary Care: Disruptive Change or Business as Usual?" *Journal of General Internal Medicine* 26, no. 8 (2011): 934–37; K. Sue Hoyt and Jean A. Proehl, "Affordable Care Act: Implications for APRNs," *Advanced Emergency Nursing Journal* 34, no. 4 (2012): 287–89.

7. Marshall et al., *Health Disparities in Appalachia;* Beth A. Bailey and Laura K. Jones Cole, "Rurality and Birth Outcomes: Findings from Southern Appalachia and the Potential Role of Pregnancy Smoking," *Journal of Rural Health* 25, no. 2 (2009): 141–49; Nengliang Yao, Stephen A. Matthews, and Marianne M. Hillemeier, "White Infant Mortality in Appalachian States, 1976–1980 and 1996–2000: Changing Patterns and Persistent Disparities," *Journal of Rural Health* 28, no. 2 (2012): 174–82.

8. Chris A. Martin et al., "Oral Health Disparities in Appalachia: Orthodontic Treatment Need and Demand," *Journal of the American Dental Association* 139, no. 5 (2008): 598–604; Marina Mileo Gorsuch, Seth G. Sanders, and Bei Wu, "Tooth Loss in Appalachia and the Mississippi Delta Relative to Other Regions in the United States, 1999–2010," *American Journal of Public Health* 104, no. 5 (2014): e85–91; Michael Hendryx, Alan M. Ducatman, Keith J. Zullig, Melissa M. Ahern, and Richard Crout, "Adult Tooth Loss for Residents of US Coal Mining and Appalachian Counties," *Community Dentistry and Oral Epidemiology* 40, no. 6 (2012): 488–97; Rebecca M. Roberts et al., "Antibiotic and Opioid Prescribing for Dental-Related Conditions in Emergency Departments: United States, 2012–2014," *Journal of the American Dental Association* 151, no. 3 (2020): 174–81.

9. H. C. Sox Jr., "Quality of Patient Care by Nurse Practitioners and Physician's Assistants: A Ten-Year Perspective," *Annals of Internal Medicine* 91, no. 3 (1979): 459–68; Sue Horrocks, Elizabeth Anderson, and Chris Salisbury, "Systematic Review of Whether Nurse Practitioners Working in Primary Care Can Provide Equivalent Care to Doctors," *British Medical Journal* 324 (2002): 819–23; M. Laurant et al., "Substitution of Doctors by Nurses in Primary Care," *Cochrane Database of Systematic Reviews* (2005): Cd001271; Ellen T. Kurtzman and Burt S. Barnow, "A Comparison of Nurse Practitioners, Physician Assistants, and Primary Care Physicians' Patterns of Practice and Quality of Care in Health Centers," *Medical Care* 55, no. 6 (2017): 615–22; Christine M. Everett, Jessica R. Schumacher, Alexandra Wright, and Maureen A. Smith, "Physician Assistants and Nurse Practitioners as a Usual Source of Care," *Journal of Rural Health* 25, no. 4 (2009): 407–14.

10. *2019 Nurse Practitioner State Practice Environment* (Arlington, VA: American Association of Nurse Practitioners, 2018), https://storage.aanp.org/www/documents/state-leg-reg/stateregulatorymap.pdf; Kaiser Family Foundation, "Nurse Practitioner Scope of Practice Laws," https://www.kff.org/other/state-indicator/total-nurse-practitioners/?currentTimeframe=0&sortModel=%7B%22colId%22:%22Location%22,%22sort%22:%22asc%22%7D; National Conference of State Legislatures, "Physician Assistants Overview," 2020, http://scopeofpracticepolicy.org/practitioners/physician-assistants/; National Conference of State Legislatures, "Nurse Practitioners Overview," 2020, http://scopeofpracticepolicy.org/practitioners/nurse-practitioners/; Kaiser Family Foundation, "Physician Assistant Scope of Practice Laws," https://www.kff.org/other/state-indicator/physician-assistant-scope-of-practice-laws/?currentTimeframe=0&sortModel=%7B%22colId%22:%22Location%22,%22sort%22:%22asc%22%7D; Margaret W. Beal, Mara E. Batzli, and Alex Hoyt, "Regulation of Certified Nurse-Midwife Scope of Practice: Change in the Professional Practice Index, 2000 to 2015," *Journal of Midwifery & Women's Health* 60, no. 5 (2015): 510–18.

11. Joanne M. Pohl, Anne Thomas, Mary Beth Bigley, and Taynin Kopanos, "Primary Care Workforce Data and the Need for Nurse Practitioner Full Practice Authority," *Health Affairs Blog,* December 13, 2018, https://www.healthaffairs.org/do/10.1377/hblog20181211.872778/full/; Linda V. Green, Sergei Savin, and Yina Lu, "Primary Care Physician Shortages Could Be Eliminated through Use of Teams, Nonphysicians, and Electronic Communication," *Health Affairs (Millwood)* 32, no. 1 (2013): 11–19; David I. Auerbach, "Will the NP Workforce Grow in the Future? New Forecasts and Implications for Healthcare Delivery," *Medical Care* 50, no. 7 (2012): 606–10; Esther Hing and Chun-Ju Hsiao, "In Which States Are Physician Assistants or Nurse Practitioners More Likely to Work in Primary Care?" *JAAPA* 28, no. 9 (2015): 46–53; Edward S. Sekscenski et al., "State Practice Environments and the Supply of Physician Assistants, Nurse Practitioners, and Certified Nurse-Midwives," *New England Journal of Medicine* 331 (1994): 1266–71; Kevin Stange, "How Does Provider Supply and Regulation Influence Health Care Markets? Evidence from Nurse Practitioners and Physician Assistants," *Journal of Health Economics* 33 (2014): 1–27; Y. Tony Yang, Laura B. Attanasio, and Katy B. Kozhimannil, "State Scope of Practice Laws, Nurse-Midwifery Workforce, and Childbirth Procedures and Outcomes," *Women's Health Issues* 26, no. 3 (2016): 262–67; Brittany L. Ranchoff and Eugene R. Declercq, "The Scope of Midwifery Practice Regulations and the Availability of the Certified Nurse-Midwifery and Certified Midwifery Workforce, 2012–2016," *Journal of Midwifery & Women's Health* 65, no. 1 (2019): 119–30.

12. Margaret Langelier et al., "Expanded Scopes of Practice for Dental Hygienists Associated with Improved Oral Health Outcomes for Adults," *Health Affairs (Millwood)* 35, no. 12 (2016): 2207–15; National Conference of State Legislators, "Oral Health Providers Overview," 2020, http://scopeofpracticepolicy.org/practitioners/oral-health-providers/.

13. Thomas C. Buchmueller, Mireille Jacobson, and Cheryl Wold, "How Far to the Hospital? The Effect of Hospital Closures on Access to Care," *Journal of Health Economics* 25, no. 4 (2006): 740–61; Andrew B. Bindman, Dennis Keane, and Nicole Lurie, "A Public Hospital Closes: Impact on Patients' Access to Care and Health Status," *JAMA* 264, no. 2 (1990): 2899–904; Margo L. Rosenbach and Debra A. Dayhoff, "Access to Care in Rural America: Impact of Hospital Closures," *Health Care Financing Review* 17, no. 1 (1995): 15–37; Morris A. Cohen and Hau L. Lee, "The Determinants of Spatial Distribution of Hospital Utilization in a Region," *Medical Care* 23, no. 1 (1985): 27–38; Harold S. Luft et al., "Does Quality Influence Choice of Hospital?" *JAMA* 263, no. 21 (1990): 2899–906; Renee Y.

Hsia and Yu-Chu Shen, "Emergency Department Closures and Openings: Spillover Effects on Patient Outcomes in Bystander Hospitals," *Health Affairs (Millwood)* 38, no. 9 (2019): 1496–504; Charleen Hsuan et al., "Ambulance Diversions Following Public Hospital Emergency Department Closures," *Health Services Research* 54, no. 4 (2019): 870–79; Charles Liu, Tanja Srebotnjak, and Renee Y. Hsia, "California Emergency Department Closures Are Associated with Increased Inpatient Mortality at Nearby Hospitals," *Health Affairs (Millwood)* 33, no. 8 (2014): 1323–29; ShinYi Chou, Mary E. Deily, and Suhui Li, "Travel Distance and Health Outcomes for Scheduled Surgery," *Medical Care* 52, no. 3 (2014): 250–57; Austin B. Frakt, "The Rural Hospital Problem," *JAMA* 321, no. 23 (2019): 2271–72; Katy B. Kozhimannil et al., "Association between Loss of Hospital-Based Obstetric Services and Birth Outcomes in Rural Counties in the United States" *JAMA* 319, no. 12 (2018): 1239–47; Richard C. Lindrooth, Marcelo C. Perraillon, Rose Y. Hardy, and Gregory J. Tung, "Understanding the Relationship between Medicaid Expansions and Hospital Closures," *Health Affairs (Millwood)* 37, no. 1 (2018): 111–20.

14. Cecil G. Sheps Center for Health Services Research, "172 Hospital Closures: January 2005–Present," 2020, https://www.shepscenter.unc.edu/programs-projects/rural-health/rural-hospital-closures/; SuZanne Troske and Alison David, *Do Hospital Closures Affect Patient Time in an Ambulance?* (Lexington: Rural and Underserved Health Research Center, University of Kentucky, 2019); Kozhimannil et al., "Association between Loss of Hospital-Based Obstetric Services"; Lindrooth et al., "Understanding the Relationship"; Chou et al., "Travel Distance and Health Outcomes"; Frakt, "Rural Hospital Problem."

15. Richard E. Doelker Jr. and Bonnie C. Bedics, "Impact of Rural Hospital Closings on the Community," *Social Work* 34, no. 6 (1989): 541–43; Richard E. McDermott, Gary C. Cornia, and Robert J. Parsons, "The Economic Impact of Hospitals in Rural Communities," *Journal of Rural Health* 7, no. 2 (1991): 117–33; George M. Holmes, Rebecca T. Slifkin, Randy K. Randolph, and Stephanie Poley, "The Effect of Rural Hospital Closures on Community Economic Health," *Health Services Research* 41, no. 2 (2006): 467–85; Mark Holmes, "Financially Fragile Rural Hospitals: Mergers and Closures," *North Carolina Medical Journal* 76, no. 1 (2015): 37–40.

16. David Dranove, Craig Garthwaite, and Christopher Ody, "Uncompensated Care Decreased at Hospitals in Medicaid Expansion States but Not at Hospitals in Nonexpansion States," *Health Affairs (Millwood)* 35, no. 8 (2016): 1471–79; David Dranove, Craig Garthwaite, and Christopher Ody, "The Impact of the ACA's Medicaid Expansion on Hospitals' Uncompensated Care Burden and the Potential Effects of Repeal," *Issue Brief (Commonwealth Fund)* 12 (2017): 1–9; Lindrooth et al., "Understanding the Relationship."

17. Balanced Budget Act of 1997, Pub. L. No. 105-33, Subtitle C: Rural Initiatives (1997); Medicare Payment Advisory Council, "Critical Access Hospitals Payment System" (2018); Michael D. Rosko and Ryan L. Mutter, "Inefficiency Differences between Critical Access Hospitals and Prospectively Paid Rural Hospitals," *Journal of Health Politics, Policy, and Law* 35, no. 1 (2010): 95–126.

18. Steven H. Woolf and Paula Braveman, "Where Health Disparities Begin: The Role of Social and Economic Determinants—and Why Current Policies May Make Matters Worse," *Health Affairs (Millwood)* 30, no. 10 (2011): 1852–59; Craig Gundersen and James P. Ziliak, "Food Insecurity and Health Outcomes," *Health Affairs (Millwood)* 34, no. 11 (2015): 1830–39; Di Zeng et al., "A Closer Look at the Rural–Urban Health Disparities: Insights from Four Major Diseases in the Commonwealth of Virginia," *Social Science and*

Medicine 140 (2015): 62–68; Traci N. Bethea et al., "The Relationship between Rural Status, Individual Characteristics, and Self-Rated Health in the Behavioral Risk Factor Surveillance System," *Journal of Rural Health* 28, no. 4 (2012): 327–38; Timothy J. Anderson, Daniel M. Saman, Martin S. Lipsky, and M. Nawal Lutfiyya, "A Cross-Sectional Study on Health Differences between Rural and Non-Rural U.S. Counties Using the County Health Rankings," *BMC Health Services Research* 15 (2015): 441.

19. E. Johnstone, "Mary Breckinridge—a Voice from the Past," *Western Journal of Nursing Research* 23, no. 6 (2001): 644–52; Nancy Schrom Dye, "Mary Breckinridge, the Frontier Nursing Service and the Introduction of Nurse-Midwifery in the United States," *Bulletin of the History of Medicine* 57, no. 4 (1983): 485–507; Anne G. Campbell, "Mary Breckinridge and the American Committee for Devastated France: The Foundations of the Frontier Nursing Service," *Register of the Kentucky Historical Society* 82, no. 3 (1984): 257–76; Marc A. Shampo and Robert A. Kyle, "Mary Breckinridge—Pioneer Nurse Brings Modern Nursing to Rural Environment," *Mayo Clinic Proceedings* 74, no. 12 (1999): 1312; Carol Crowe-Carraco, "Mary Breckinridge and the Frontier Nursing Service," *Register of the Kentucky Historical Society* 76, no. 3 (1978): 179–91.

20. Dye, "Mary Breckinridge."

21. Crowe-Carraco, "Mary Breckinridge."

22. Johnstone, "Mary Breckinridge"; Dye, "Mary Breckinridge"; Campbell, "Mary Breckinridge"; Shampo and Kyle, "Mary Breckinridge"; Crowe-Carraco, "Mary Breckinridge"; G. Issacs, "The Frontier Nursing Service: Family Nursing in Rural Areas," *Clinical Obstetrics and Gynecology* 15, no. 2 (1972): 394–407.

23. Crowe-Carraco, "Mary Breckinridge"; Frontier Nursing University, "Distance Education," 2019, https://frontier.edu/student-experience/distance-education/; Frontier Nursing University, "Frontier Nursing University—a Journey through Time," https://frontier.edu/about-frontier/history/.

24. "Transforming Rural Health Care: Appalachian Regional Healthcare," *Nursing Administration Quarterly* 23, no. 1 (1998): 41–61; Richard C. Smoot, "Medical History Notes from Appalachia," *Appalachian Review* 23, no. 4 (1995): 21–28; "Operations under the UMWA Welfare and Retirement Fund," *Monthly Labor Review* 77, no. 11 (1954): 1232–34; Robert J. Myers, "Further Experience of the UMWA Welfare and Retirement Fund," *Industrial & Labor Relations Review* (1961): 556–62, https://doi.org/10.1177/001979396101400404.

25. "Transforming Rural Health Care"; Smoot, "Medical History Notes"; Appalachian Regional Healthcare, "Appalachian Regional Healthcare: About Us," 2019, http://www.arh.org/about_us.aspx.

26. J. Cheeves, "The Face of Poverty Never Escaped His Moment of Fame," *Lexington Herald-Leader,* November 16, 2013, https://www.kentucky.com/news/special-reports/fifty-years-of-night/article44453805.html; Appalachian Regional Development Act of 1965, 40 U.S.C. Subtitle IV §141–3.

27. PARC, *Appalachia: A Report by the President's Commission on Appalachia* (Washington, DC: PARC, 1964); An Act to Mobilize the Human and Financial Resources of the Nation to Combat Poverty in the United States, Pub. L. No. 88-452 (1964); Martha J. Bailey and Andrew Goodman-Bacon, "The War on Poverty's Experiment in Public Medicine: Community Health Centers and the Mortality of Older Americans," *American Economic Review* 105, no. 3 (2015): 1067–104.

28. Appalachian Regional Development Act of 1965.

29. Alison F. Davis et al., *Program Evaluation of the Appalachian Regional Commission's Health Projects, 2004–2010* (Washington, DC: Appalachian Regional Commission, 2015), https://www.arc.gov/wp-content/uploads/2020/06/ProgramEvaluationofARCsHealthProjects2004-2010.pdf.

30. PDA and Sheps Center, *Health Care Costs;* Halverson et al., *Analysis of Disparities;* Marshall et al., *Health Disparities in Appalachia.*

31. Ian T. MacQueen et al., "Recruiting Rural Healthcare Providers Today: A Systematic Review of Training Program Success and Determinants of Geographic Choices," *Journal of General Internal Medicine* 33, no. 2 (2018): 191–99; Vernon Curran and James Rourke, "The Role of Medical Education in the Recruitment and Retention of Rural Physicians," *Medical Teacher* 26, no. 3 (2004): 265–72; Carolyn M. Pepper, Ryan H. Sandefer, and Matt J. Gray, "Recruiting and Retaining Physicians in Very Rural Areas," *Journal of Rural Health* 26, no. 2 (2010): 196–200; Puja Verma et al., "A Systematic Review of Strategies to Recruit and Retain Primary Care Doctors," *BMC Health Services Research* 16 (2016): 126; Donald L. Pathman et al., "Medical Training Debt and Service Commitments: The Rural Consequences," *Journal of Rural Health* 16, no. 3 (2000): 264–72.

32. Daniel G. Mareck, "Federal and State Initiatives to Recruit Physicians to Rural Areas," *AMA Journal of Ethics* 13, no. 5 (2011): 304–9; Health Resources and Services Administration, "State Loan Repayment Program Grantee Awards Map," 2020, https://nhsc.hrsa.gov/loan-repayment/state-loan-repayment-program/map.

7

The Appalachian Environment

Alan Ducatman and Rachel E. Dixon

The Appalachian environment is sculpted by humans in ways that affect the health of its inhabitants. In large swaths of Appalachia, especially in Central Appalachian "coal country," sustainable economic success and environmentally healthy living have proved elusive. This is unsurprising: it has been known for decades that environmental degradation does not attract residential wealth and that low socioeconomic status predicts both environmental and health risk. Students of public health study these intersections in courses on "environmental justice." The colorful, potentially pejorative journalistic term for these places is "sacrifice zone." Yet labeling Appalachia a sacrifice zone is a misleading and pessimistic generalization. Problematic conditions are not uniform. Further, where they exist, they are partially reversible and certainly addressable, given political will and planning.

This chapter explores issues of environmental health and environmental justice in the Appalachian region, providing historical context for and current examples of links between health outcomes and environmental factors. Wherever possible, it shows that the region retains natural advantages and that existing problems stem in part from human assumptions that can be altered and problematic decisions that can be addressed (such as ratepayer costs and health consequences of overreliance on fossil fuels). Improvements can be achieved, even in the most problematic areas. Envisioning the environment and its needs as an essential part of the infrastructure will materially assist the process.

The United States has experienced decades of historic economic attainment, and the Appalachian economy has absorbed some of this success. Today, *only* around 16 percent of the region still experiences the most abject poverty, meaning that rural poverty is neither monolithic nor historically inevitable in Appalachia. It is the case, however, that large parts of the region are accelerating toward poverty. The map of Appalachian poverty, in areas experiencing the most consistent and ongoing population loss, bears some resemblance to a map of the region's most valuable mineral resources. Coal country is afflicted by air pollution, water pollution, population loss, and something else: the absence of sufficient planned infrastructure to sustain development on a rough mountain landscape. In the less densely populated areas of Appalachia, notably in Central Appalachian coal country, the population continues its long decline, in striking contrast to most other parts of the United States.[1]

The "coal camp" or "coal town" illustrates why considering the overarch-ing concept of built environment is valuable to the understanding of human health. The coal camp was a workplace and a deliberately unsustainable resi-dential development: a home with insufficient infrastructure for community living, with rich social affiliations and economic conflicts. It was a means to provide housing that was implicitly not intended for long-term development. It was a social unit with its own internal governance and norms that ensured an indebted workforce organized around an extractive economy. At the same time, it was a source of substantial environmental degradation. Today, the coal towns are vanishing or gone, but their legacy of insufficient infrastructure and environmental consequences remains. The lessons of more than a century of coal dominance and deliberate inattention to sustainability—whether learned, never learned, or forgotten—will not become less important as the dominance of coal power is shared with or replaced by other industries.

The Ambient and Built Environment: Extraction in the Absence of Economic Development

A confluence of geographic, political, legal, and historical factors has impeded coordinated, long-term regional development in "official" Appalachia. As explained in chapter 2, Appalachia covers all of one state (West Virginia) and parts of twelve others; this region is defined by the Appalachian Regional Commission (ARC), a federally supported economic development agency. The difference between the broader geographic region and the narrower "official" population is important and instructive: New England and eastern Canada share the mountains (and many of the problems) of the thirteen Appalachian states, but they have fewer natural resources and have generally been more successful in addressing environmental health issues and combating poverty. Thus, comparisons with non-ARC counties in states that include the Appala-chian Mountains are explicitly intended to show that different approaches to sustainability are possible. The point is that the low population densities, espe-cially in Central Appalachia (62.7 inhabitants per square mile), and the high rates of economically distressed and economically threatened counties (more than 45 percent of Appalachian counties) have nonrandom causes, including causes that can be addressed.

Geology and Geography

Geology and geography interact to affect Appalachian health and economic well-being, in part because economic life in the mountains has increased exposure to natural disasters and complicated regional planning efforts. The history is not limited to fossil fuels. For example, the consequences of one early industry—timber production—illustrate the challenges, the planning complexity, and the potential reversibility of poor health outcomes. Appalachian timber (including from non-ARC regions in New England) built eastern US cities and suburbs in the nineteenth and early twentieth centuries. Much of Appalachia was completely or nearly completely deforested, with many consequences. Historically, large uncontrolled forest fires in Appalachia started from left-behind timber in logged-over areas. A century ago, the region had few civic means to police, prevent, or fight fires in logged-over rural areas. More than 1.7 million acres of West Virginia burned in 1907 alone. Runoff caused by deforestation and forest fires in logged-over areas was so severe a century ago that the quality of surface water was threatened by its silt burden.[2]

The seldom-recounted history of deforestation provides evidence that challenges in the Appalachian environment are not unique to currently dominant industries such as coal and natural gas. It also demonstrates that problems are at least partially reversible. Today, scientific forest management practices are in place, and forest fires and runoff represent diminished but still potent threats. This threat is due to the more extensive understory and diminished water-holding properties of second-growth forests and their soils. Diminished topsoil coverage occurs after fires and runoff, and it takes centuries to fully rebound. The more valuable, deep-rooted tree species have trouble competing on these diminished soils. (Progress toward soil recovery must also account for introduced forest pests and climate change; these problems are not unique to Appalachia but may have outsized effects in the extensive Appalachian forests.) Yet the more important and optimistic point is that forests and health are improving over time—these problems are tractable to good governance and planned solutions.[3]

Although fire is still common and natural, large-scale fires have mostly receded from memory. However, the possibility that a large-scale fire could recur is an important planning problem, as drought could cause massive fires in the region once more. National firefighting capabilities have greatly improved, but lessons related to building fire-resistant residential communities in heavily forested areas are not yet routinely implemented in the region.

Appalachian Mountain counties that are outside of ARC-served boundaries have faced similar issues, yet they have overcome them more quickly and with better results through strong leadership. Vermont's forests, like those elsewhere in the Appalachian mountain chain, had been 80 percent deforested by the end of the nineteenth century. Just as in nineteenth-century ARC Appalachia, Vermont wood products supported the growth of distant cities and provided local employment. However, influential nineteenth-century reformers began to advocate against the Vermont timber harvest, noting that it was unsustainable for employment purposes and a source of soil erosion that threatened the state's water resources. Railroad entrepreneur Frederick Billings (for whom Billings, Montana, is named) demonstrated, on his own land, that Vermonters could make a living in dairy farming, which in turn led to the active reforestation of hillsides that were too steep for dairy use. This successful demonstration was widely copied and played a role in transforming the Vermont economy to one that subsequently featured a century of successful dairy production. After several decades of dairy price volatility, Vermont entrepreneurs have again diversified, sending niche farm-to-table products to regional cities. This transformation is also beginning in counties within ARC's service area that are close to major cities, but cultivation of and investment in regional farm products are still far less common in Appalachia than in the hills and valleys of New England.[4]

Further, environmental decisions are arguably more complex in ARC states than in states like Vermont, owing in large part to the dominance of coal, oil, and gas extraction. Policy makers in the region have to cope with mounting poverty as a result of numerous abandoned (and a few operating) underground mines and under- or unrehabilitated surface mines (strip mines). Today, surface mining has reemerged with new technology and new consequences for the built environment. In the absence of easily accessible coal, modern mining techniques target coal that is hundreds of feet beneath the surface, creating massive "mountaintop removal" projects to reach seams. Although the large-scale blasting and industrial earthmoving processes needed to excise mountaintops create jobs during production, they pose several challenges to local communities. First, blasting and removing an entire mountaintop generates substantial particulate air pollution (dust). Second, the practice can decimate livable landscapes. Though some "rehabilitated" former mine sites are suitable for golf courses, prisons, strip malls, roads, or runways, the majority have limited economic potential and remain undeveloped sources of ongoing contamination. Long-term ecological outcomes include loss of biodiversity and a legacy of water pollution. Water runs off the surface through mine rubble ("valley fill") and encounters minerals and organics that can affect water quality for generations. Polluted runoff, whether from underground or surface mines, is long lasting. It can be extremely expensive to bring in water from alternative sources because it may have to be pumped uphill and across mountain ridges. To obtain potable water, then, residents must subsidize expensive solutions to problems caused by mining. Federal reclamation programs seek to regulate closed mines, but they are underfunded (by billions of dollars) and often ineffective in dealing with the thousands of sites.[5]

Politics and Industry Power

Even where the environment is relatively pristine, new developments often lack the normal infrastructure that would be expected in much of the rest of the nation, such as sidewalks, storm-water runoff capture, or roads with developed shoulders and space for passing. The poster child for infrastructure underdevelopment in Appalachia is the "straight pipe," a euphemism for the situation in which sewage flows from a dwelling or work site straight into the nearest stream. Although this practice is becoming less common, it persists in many areas. There are several reasons why straight pipes are still in use. First and foremost, local officials are wary of putting too much pressure on home and business owners for noncompliance with sanitary codes, lest they lose even more residents in economically marginal and impoverished, depopulated counties. In addition, the shift from federal to state funding for wastewater treatment projects disproportionately affects poor communities. Shifting costs onto landholders may seem reasonable in wealthier neighborhoods in other regions, but it may be less viable in poorer regions. The reality is that water flows downhill from the mountains, so the millions who rely on the James, New, Potomac, Roanoke, Shenandoah, Tennessee, Ohio, and other river systems with Appalachian headwaters must inevitably consider the meaning of shared resources. The persistence of straight pipes should be seen in the context of the bigger picture of insufficient resources for regional development and underfunding of water utility operators.[6]

This absence of policy decisions contributes to the fragmented nature of Appalachian development. This is perhaps best exemplified by the relationship between the coal industry and economic planning. Coal mining became the dominant industry in Appalachia after the Civil War. Today, a residual, highly mechanized, and greatly downsized Appalachian coal industry is tenuously hanging on, with ongoing economic and environmental consequences. It struggles for profitability and supports far fewer jobs than it did even a decade ago. In West Virginia, there were fewer than 20,000 coal jobs in 2018, and at least seven mines have closed since the last employment report. (A smaller metallurgical coal industry is somewhat more economically robust than coal mined for power generation.) Throughout coal country, industry leaders have fostered an elitist "war on coal" narrative to explain the industry's decline, which regional planners and elected officials have parroted. This rhetoric portrays the decline as the result of something other than simple capitalist forces, and it implies that coal mining is the victim of arbitrarily imposed policies from outside the region. This rhetoric may serve public relations needs when there are ongoing layoffs and the first losses are miners' pensions. However, there is little chance that the rhetoric will alter the future of energy planning, because less expensive sources of energy are available, independent of the rhetoric. Nevertheless, the destructive "war on coal" rhetoric dominates regional policy, stalls regional planning, and diminishes economic innovation.

Big lies grow from smaller narratives that contain kernels of truth. For example, leaders of the Appalachian coal industry can legitimately say that coal has been unfairly singled out as a contributor to climate change in comparison to natural gas. All fossil fuels release climate-forcing pollutants; however, federal policies of the last decade have incorrectly stated that coal is creating more greenhouse warming than the competing and relatively less expensive natural gas. To reach this conclusion, federal policy considered one part of the energy cycle—the actual power generated—measured in British thermal units (BTUs). Per BTU, coal releases about 50 percent more carbon dioxide than natural gas. However, this calculation is scientifically incomplete. The federal climate change approach, portraying natural gas as a "bridge" to a better future, underestimates the greenhouse effects of massive (but more difficult to measure) releases of methane and other volatile gases at every stage of natural gas recovery. Research has clarified that methane releases are both far greater and far more climate-damaging than policy makers acknowledged when espousing natural gas as a better alternative to coal. Thus, the coal industry's concern that natural gas has gotten an undeserved pass has some legitimacy. However, that concern is largely unrelated to the "war on coal" rhetoric, which deliberately fails to call public attention to the consequences of reliance on fossil fuels.[7]

A less-publicized concern of the coal industry is differential business severance taxes in some states. A lower tax on gas production compared with coal production is an inexplicable policy puzzle for future voters who are told that the gas industry will somehow manage to build infrastructure and pay for environmental rehabilitation without paying development taxes to offset its wide-ranging societal costs. Rebalancing the tax structure will not begin to address the cost differences that have led to the rapid ascendance of gas as a less expensive source of fossil fuel energy in the United States and internationally, independent of local taxation quirks. The "war on coal" narrative has been successful, in the sense that it influences policy and asserts regional dominance. However, it cannot bring back a diminishing industry because it conveniently ignores current capitalist realities based on accessible resources and consumer costs.[8]

Coal country is rich in natural gas, with attendant infrastructure problems that may be less discussed than those related to coal. The US oil and natural gas industry began in Appalachia in the nineteenth century, and the most easily accessible resources were exhausted by the early twentieth century. Thanks to new technologies, gas production is now outpacing regional coal production.

The technical developments that have enabled access to new sources of natural gas include the ability to drill deep wells that can laterally follow gas-bearing rocks over long distances. Vast quantities of water are introduced at high pressure to hydrofracture the rock and release the trapped gas ("fracking"). Yet the success of this technology hides serious problems, including environmental risks that are exacerbated by questionable profitability and sustainability. In large swaths of coal country, gas rigs now dot the landscape and interrupt the forest cover.

The production of natural gas unencumbered by regional planning has led to a substantial reliance on nonregional labor and the generation of excess capacity, greatly exceeding regional needs and resulting in a lowering of natural gas prices below profitability. This is best considered the squandering of a potentially valuable resource. To address the glut, the industry has proposed numerous natural gas pipelines to transport resources out of Appalachia for use in the wider United States, Canada, and beyond. These pipelines are far from innocuous to neighbors. Compressor stations that pull the gas along the pipeline routes can be constant sources of noise, similar to the roar of jet engines. The pipelines themselves are especially difficult to build and maintain safely in the steep Appalachian terrain, where thin soils tend to run off easily and buried hillside pipelines are susceptible to soil slips and catastrophic pipeline failure. In Appalachia, evidence of poor pipeline construction practices causing hillside erosion and stream degradation have led to de minimis fines for flagrant violations of regulations. The installers consider these small fines a cost of doing business.[9]

Potentially valuable secondary products that rely on natural gas production, such as ethane for plastic products, are being sold at low prices or simply wasted due to a glut. The rush to development has consistently sent gas to market before there is a regional capacity to create value-added products, and it is possible that the region will never develop a sustainable value-added coordination. Instead, based on legal precedents and the preferences of elected officials, short-term economic goals and the perceived needs of mineral-rights owners have dominated, while attempts to use nonrenewable resources in ways that encourage permanent development remain a hope.

Law

Legal quirks constrain long-term regional development and combine with the political pull of industry to favor short-term gain. The "split estate"—the legal severing of underground mineral rights from surface rights—is just one example. Under a split estate, landowners can sell the mineral rights to their property while keeping the surface rights. Their heirs can further subdivide the rights over generations. Over time, it is possible that only a minority of the owners of underground rights will reside near the land in question. Numerous variations of the split estate exist to separate those with an economic incentive to care about the land itself from those who can decide how the land will be used if there are valuable minerals under the surface. Consequences outlast the lifetimes of industrial activity and corporate entities, marring the built environment and guaranteeing the absence of funds for remediation. This problem has plagued Appalachian coal extraction for more than a century, and it is being recapitulated with the reemergence of natural gas production.[10]

The legacy of split estates and a short-term focus on jobs at any cost is a lack of stewardship. Resources are accessed and depleted in the absence of plans to develop sustainable industry and with no consideration of the resources needed to remediate environmental damage.

The poorest parts of Appalachia struggle with problems that are not always visible from the road. Citizens in other parts of the country may be unable to imagine damage to homes and businesses from the eventual collapse of abandoned underground mines, yet that is a very real possibility. Abandoned gas wells are a similar invisible hazard. Many were not required to be "capped" (engineered to fully close their conduits) and became a source of gas intrusion into nearby residential water wells and indoor air pollution in nearby homes. Pennsylvania alone has more than 25,000 abandoned oil and gas wells with no apparent owner, and that does not take into account the innumerable abandoned wells whose locations are unknown. Hotly debated is how often the new type of unconventional gas well has created the same problem for nearby residents. The homeowner and gas well–operator narratives are quite different, and the burden of proving lost value has been on the homeowner.

There is neither the funding nor the political will to prioritize these problems. When Pennsylvania required one corporate owner to cap abandoned wells, the owner's response was that the mineral rights of the closed wells had been sold to distant third parties. The owner made the additional thought-provoking claim that the requirement could not be met in any case because industry resources were limited and there were too few competent vendors capable of plugging abandoned wells. That defense implies that the work cannot be done because no one is doing it, despite the massive numbers of closed wells that need to be capped.[11]

Lack of Infrastructure

Transportation is yet another challenge that adds to Appalachians' disadvantage and ill health. Intractable problems related to the development of mountainous terrain are exacerbated in Appalachia by historical underfunding of highway infrastructure and regional tolerance of poorly engineered roads. In the nineteenth and early twentieth centuries, railroads that climbed around or tunneled through the Appalachian Mountains linked Appalachian timber and coal resources with eastern markets. This fostered the tradition of American engineering. Road development is logically another boon to rural areas, as the reach of roads can greatly exceed the reach of railroads. Yet road building has been less advantageous in the Appalachian region.

The lag in funding for highways in the mountains of Appalachia is related to a circular problem of low population density in rural areas and the high cost of mountain highway development and maintenance. Further, Appalachian development has often been relegated to last place in federal highway man-dates. The Appalachian Regional Development Act of 1965 finally authorized funds for Appalachian highway development, long after federal highways served the rest of the nation. For example, US Interstate 68 linked metropolitan Washington, DC, with Central Appalachia only in 1991; western expansion into Appalachian Ohio is desperately needed but not yet begun. The existing road lacks merging on- and off-ramps to secondary roads in places where pop-ulation growth has been fostered, leading to foreseeable traffic snarls that limit the beneficial economic impact in developing cities along the way.

Underdeveloped highway systems compound the challenges of year-round life in mountainous terrain, affecting many aspects of rural living. Local schools have consolidated due to population loss, forcing students to endure long-distance bus commutes on hazardous mountain roads. For simple eco-nomic reasons, most Appalachian states have ceased to honor the ostensible time limits on school bus rides for children. For the entire population, limited road development has had a measurable impact on public health, including higher transportation mortality rates that are only partly explained by the region's rural nature.[12]

Research from the University of North Carolina confirms another irony of living in a rural mountain landscape: these small communities can be "highly unwalkable," with a general absence of sidewalks, road shoulders, and bicycle lanes. Clinicians are aware of the irony of recommending that their rural patients drive to the nearest shopping mall to walk for exercise. Obesity is substantially more prevalent in Appalachia than in the rest of the United States (31.0 percent versus 27.1 percent in 2012), with a particular concentration in Central Appala-chia (34.7 percent). Absence of exercise is a contributing risk factor to the devel-opment of diabetes. Researchers from East Tennessee State University note the presence of a "diabetes belt" in Central and Southern Appalachian counties.[13]

These obvious deficiencies in the built environment are seldom linked to policy and planning opportunities, yet such problems are addressable. And there are economic payoffs from building highways and creating pedestrian access: mayors and business groups in large and small Appalachian cities have credited greenway and trail development with improving local economic activity. Nevertheless, developers' opposition to something as simple as requiring sidewalks often hamstrings Appalachian development policy.[14]

Air Quality

Six decades of steady environmental progress have markedly improved air quality in the United States, including throughout Appalachia. External comparisons can provide perspective: Air quality in the most polluted regions of the United States is generally far better than in industrialized or urban areas of developing countries. Furthermore, death rates and morbidity from air pollution are far lower in all parts of the United States compared with low- and middle-income countries (such as China and India) and with parts of Southeast Asia. There are also important limitations and opportunities for improvement. Progress in reducing air pollution has been less substantial in much of Appalachia compared with the rest of the United States. Explanations include natural phenomena, overreliance on coal, shortsighted opposition to renewable energy development, and ongoing regional disdain for the enforcement of regulations, seemingly based on the belief that tolerance of air pollution fosters employment. As a result, regional policy decisions and leadership attitudes have pushed state watchdog agencies into ambiguous and compromised positions in the eyes of local communities.[15]

Natural phenomena can complicate efforts to improve the air quality in Appalachia. Weather conditions over steep topography favor local temperature inversions, trapping a layer of cold air under warmer air in the valleys. Temperature inversions are most common and intense in the fall and early winter, when wood burning is a common home-heating supplement. The inversion layer can last for hours to days. The science of how natural phenomena and man-made pollution interact is illustrated by an episode in Donora, Pennsylvania, a small (current population less than 5,000) industrial city on the banks of the Monongahela River, about twenty miles south of Pittsburgh. It houses a small museum with an intriguing theme: "Clean Air Started Here." It did, and it started badly. During a temperature inversion in the fall of 1948, a thick, blinding "fog" trapped the acid particulates emitted from the local steel mills and zinc wire mills. Today, that fog would be called "smog," and it would be considered a public health emergency. However, in 1948, smog events during temperature inversions—which trap the pollution below a layer of cold air—were a common and accepted part of life in mill towns. The Donora museum's website has photographs of typical air pollution episodes, with streetlamps illuminating dusk-like conditions during the daytime. The

1948 event resulted in twenty acute or subacute fatalities and entered the national consciousness; it was followed by at least a decade of elevated respiratory mortality. The Donora story recapitulated earlier and deadlier events in Belgium's industrialized Meuse Valley and in London, England. Air quality improvements began immediately and were coordinated in the United States, including across Appalachia following the establishment of the Environmental Protection Agency in 1970 during the Nixon administration.[16]

Appreciation for air pollution's effect on human health increased in the 1970s when Harvard University's "Six Cities" study evaluated mortality and other health-related outcomes from air pollution in six cities, including two in Appalachia. Cities as large as St. Louis, Missouri, and Topeka, Kansas, had less measurable air pollution than the small city of Steubenville, Ohio. Steubenville, home to professional athletes, military leaders, and famous entertainers, grew around its paper mills, nail factories, and steel mills. Today, energy and utility industries (and affiliated consultants) publicly question the findings from the Six Cities study because the data were collected in an era before deidentification permitted ethical sharing. This approach is part of the "war on coal" narrative and has been used in temporarily successful ploys to diminish air pollution control standards. Scientifically, the narrative cannot hold up because it ignores the more substantive point that the findings were independently and repeatedly confirmed using exposure measures and health outcomes from other populations in the United States and from around the world, including new health outcomes that were not uncovered by the original study.[17]

There are more than 36,000 references to air pollution and health in the US National Library of Medicine, extending the effects of air pollution to respiratory and nonrespiratory mortality and diverse morbidities of many types, including cardiovascular disease, cancer, neurologic disease, and reproductive issues. It is certain that air pollution—whether measured as particulate matter, nitrogen oxides, sulfur oxides, ozone, or a host of specific workplace contaminants—causes disease and that improvements in air pollution increase life expectancy. Nevertheless, elected officials and some appointed policy makers in Appalachia have pushed the narrative that improving air quality is part of the "war on coal." Appalachians have tolerated years of casual enforcement of local pollution controls, seemingly based on the false hope that relaxing air pollution standards will stimulate regional economic investment. The reality is that air pollution has consequences in Appalachia, and the push for lax enforcement and tolerance of diminished air quality have not attracted new business investment.[18]

Air pollution therefore poses a health risk across the Appalachian Mountain region that seems unnecessary, based on the lower population density, and should be reversible. The recent history of Appalachia's most populous metropolitan area illustrates both national progress and ongoing regional problems. Pittsburgh's metropolitan region includes parts of Ohio and West Virginia. Today, its air quality is remarkably better than it was before the 1940s and 1950s. Like Donora, Pittsburgh's history includes inversion events characterized as "midday darkness." Improvement in the city's air quality is unquestioned, but so is the residual problem. Among the more than 200 US metropolitan regions, Pittsburgh still ranks as one of the worst for air pollution (seventh worst in one ranking), especially for small particulate matter known as PM 2.5 (particles measuring less than 2.5 microns), which can easily get into the deepest parts of the respiratory system and do the most damage. The trend in metropolitan Pittsburgh worsened recently, and this cannot be attributed to the absence of technology to fight air pollution or to population density. The extended Pittsburgh metropolitan area has about 440 residents per square mile and is growing more slowly than most US metropolitan areas. Even New York City, with its 5,600 inhabitants per square mile, enjoys better air quality. This is a problem in many parts of Appalachia and is one explanation for poor health outcomes in the region.[19]

Microscale air pollution from specific industrial sources is seldom measured and seriously underreported, disempowering residents. The reemergence of massive surface coal mining through mountaintop removal has added significant amounts of dust particulates to the immediate environment. Satellite evidence from rural Virginia has also documented that air quality along coal-carrying truck routes can be seriously impacted. A review of air quality reporting data in ARC counties reveals that many do not take actual measurements from within their own counties. Instead, public health agencies rely on surrogate measures from neighboring counties, some of which have only a single, central monitoring station. Despite the obvious need, there is a paucity of funding to detect health outcomes related to point sources of pollution in Appalachia. To the extent that research has already documented adverse health outcomes, this is discouraging. Studies of health outcomes near surface mining activity have shown an excess of undesirable effects, including but not limited to birth defects, heart disease, and respiratory disease. These findings are consistent with what has long been accepted as the consequence of exposure to air pollution in populations everywhere, yet the information still seems to be controversial in Appalachia, and there is insufficient funding for further robust study.[20]

There is a parallel need for information about air pollution near the numerous shale gas operations in the region. Where reports exist, sporadic measurements above acceptable levels have been reported from wellheads. The impact of industrial vehicular traffic around unconventional natural gas pads is also of interest. Shale gas extraction can involve thousands of heavy truck visits per pad (about 10,000 heavy truck trips during the life of a well). Findings, so far, are that residents living nearby have experienced an increase in self-reported symptoms, as well as measurable outcomes such as endocrine disruption and lower birth weights. Air pollution is not the only concern; noise and light pollution may be just as important to the health and disordered sleep of residents. Efforts to characterize and monitor these effects have come from university researchers, but few if any public health entities are systematically addressing problems related to natural resource extraction in Appalachia.[21]

Residents living near problematic point sources of pollution may only have access to misleading data obtained from sources more than thirty miles and several mountain ridges away. The ongoing conversation about whether known sources of air pollution actually contribute to poor health outcomes in Appalachia is unscientific, and this has real health consequences. The absence of air pollution measures may reflect two regional beliefs: the health effects of air pollution are not pertinent to the people of Appalachia, or the inhabitants are better off economically if exposures and outcomes are unknown. Unwillingness to police local sources of air pollution and overreliance on industry goals (including overuse of fossil fuels) are seldom considered when regional health outcomes are discussed. That is unfortunate, because these factors can be addressed, and there is reason to be optimistic about both problems. Consumers will seek inexpensive energy and cleaner air, and misleading rhetoric will eventually succumb to opportunity.[22]

Water Quality

Water may be the most valuable and overlooked natural resource in Appalachia. The region is blessed with naturally renewable river and stream surface water and abundant groundwater. Large areas of Appalachia will continue to have access to potentially potable water resources even as other regions face increasing water scarcity due to population pressure and climate change. However, many Appalachian water resources are only *potentially* potable because they contain pollutants from past and ongoing industrial sources. Water-related barriers to regional economic development are numerous: an expensive legacy of fouled water sources, ongoing unsustainable and poorly regulated extractive industrial practices, insufficient wastewater and storm-water runoff infrastructure, and insufficient attention to reclamation. Yet these hurdles are surmountable and could provide enormous economic opportunity if they were prioritized by policy makers.

Despite these problems, there have been some important successes. Virtually all of Appalachia has long had access to modern indoor plumbing. Municipal sewage treatment and industrial pretreatments have greatly improved, although they are still far from where they need to be. In addition, some streams that were rendered uninhabitable for most aquatic species by coal-waste runoff or chemical pollutants have been returned by various means to the point where they can sustain a successful game-fish industry. Investment that supports renewable resource tourism has also encouraged regional development, especially in the Blue Ridge and Great Smoky Mountain regions. Water quality in the extensive national forest headwaters, in particular, is high, even near urban areas. All these things represent major advantages and gains.[23]

Yet important challenges persist. In much of Appalachian coal country, the water running from abandoned mines and coal-waste dump sites leaves an orange stain on streamside rocks, sometimes called "poverty stones." The orange stain originates from the mineral wastes, such as iron sulfides and iron oxides, of underground and surface mines. These minerals gradually deposit their acidic burden, with its sickly color, on the rocky soil of Appalachia. Aluminum, arsenic, boron, cadmium, copper, manganese, mercury, and selenium may also be present in undesirable quantities. The drainage can render streams uninhabitable for susceptible amphibian, fish, and aquatic mammal species. Coal burning is an additional atmospheric source of soil and water pollution. The volatilized mercury from burning coal settles back on the land over broad areas. This is the primary (but not the only) source of mercury pollution in freshwater fish in the United States, especially in Appalachia. Coal burning also produces substantial quantities of ash that must be disposed of. Some of the ash is spread on roads, along with salt, for winter ice control, adding to the mineral waste and pH burden of coal country's water. Some of this waste ash can be incorporated into useful products such as drywall, but the supply greatly exceeds the demand. Ash heaps dot the Appalachian landscape near coal-burning facilities. They are sometimes (but not always) protected by a thin layer of grass-covered soil. Ash dumps sometimes collapse, and ash containment ponds can escape their banks, leading to massive pollution such as occurred in Tennessee's Clinch River and in the western Carolina Piedmont in 2014.

The most common and regionally unique problem is clogging of the subsurface "French" water drains designed to keep homes and businesses dry. Pyrite-laden water from coal mines produces an acid grit that dissolves structural foundation gravel. This clogs the French drains, causing interior flooding. These inherited, residual problems of energy production in Central Appalachia are preventable with proper zoning, investment, regulation, remediation, and planning—but they are too rarely considered during the development phase. This is a classic example of the kind of costs borne by homeowners because energy producers are not expected to bear the after-use costs of their activities. Operations routinely close without full remediation or assets to address the long-term and fully predictable environmental costs. Federal funds set aside to clean up acid mine drainage are inadequate to address even 1 percent of the residual problem.

Coal slurry is a source of water pollution that results from the beneficial control of coal-related air pollution. Coal burning generates far less air pollution in the United States than in many other parts of the world because the coal is of a higher quality, and it is generally "cleaned" by a sophisticated water- and chemical-based treatment process at or near the mine. It is then transported elsewhere for fuel production and "dewatered" before being used for power generation. The cleaning process creates massive quantities of viscous coal "slurry." This waste is stored in slurry "ponds" behind containment dams, which are just large, chemical-laden lakes. The 1972 Buffalo Creek dam failure created a thirty-foot flood crest of viscous black water, killing 125 people and displacing more than 4,000. The dam had just been inspected and deemed safe. The official disaster report pointed out an obvious trade-off: the beneficial coal cleaning created coal slurry ponds fraught with environmental hazards. A similar disaster in Martin County, Kentucky, killed all the wildlife in headwater creeks of the Tug Fork and Big Sandy Rivers in 2000.[24]

Although cleaning coal protects air quality, slurry ponds adversely affect water quality, even when they work as intended. The dammed coal-waste pond is a way station along a natural stream, and the dam releases the natural stream, carrying industrial pollutants, at a controlled rate. In addition, sediment settling creates permanently polluted bottomland along the stream's path. Unfortunately, alternatives to this disposal method are not obvious, and the practice persists. The waste pond is not the only place where the air–water pollution trade-off occurs. Water is used to "scrub" coal-burning power plants' smokestacks, successfully reducing the emissions of several kinds of air pollutants. However, this water, with its residual burden of new pollutants, is then returned to the lake or stream source once the scrubbing is completed.

Wastewater from natural gas hydrofracturing creates similar problems on a smaller scale. Holding ponds for "returned water" have impermanent plastic linings, so pollution will eventually be released to deeper soil. In addition, the mishandling of surface "flowback water" has created local problems. Elevated levels of diesel-range organic pollutants in groundwater near the Marcellus gas operations are thought to be derived mainly from surface activities rather than well-casing failures and the deep transfer of contaminants. The well operator can reduce the costs of purchasing water and using tanker trucks when the hydrofracturing water can be obtained directly from a local stream. However, such stream withdrawals can threaten the flow of small local streams in summer, causing additional concerns about wildlife and increasing downstream sedimentation.

Today, much of the returned water is reused and eventually, when it is no longer usable, trucked off-site and reinjected into a disposal well. This decreases the amount of surface pollution if it is done correctly. A future concern related to this activity is induced seismicity; this has already been experienced in other hydro-fracturing regions, but so far, it has not been a problem in Appalachia.[25]

There are other longer-term worries about current gas-related activities. As exhausted wells are capped and then abandoned, it is unclear whether new casing failures might lead to long-term sources of contamination for future generations. In addition, it is already known that stray gas can find its way into local residents' well water. Homeowners' experience of this problem is instructive for understanding environmental justice issues and cost externality. When pollution has been discovered in well water, drilling-site owners have routinely pointed out that the homeowners have no proof that recent industrial activity is the source of that pollution; because the homeowners have not performed chain-of-custody advance testing, the existence of an earlier source of pollution cannot be disproved (ironically, past drilling activity is most commonly blamed). Historically, new drilling operations were permitted to commence without requiring drillers to obtain chain-of-custody sampling and secure storage of neighboring water sources—the same information homeowners cannot produce. This common legal defense illustrates the economic burdens placed on homeowners who live next to one of the thousands of point sources of this burgeoning industry in Central Appalachia. So far, policy makers have not addressed concerns related to this new activity.[26]

Industrial hog farming affects water quality (in addition to causing odor and health concerns) in smaller areas of ARC states, such as in North Carolina and neighboring Virginia. For several reasons, industrial-scale hog-confinement agriculture is environmentally and economically problematic, and the costs of water pollution have clearly been underestimated.[27]

Although it seems obvious, regional policy makers and regulatory authorities routinely overlook the fact that surface and underground water polluted by runoff from mines, waste ponds, and ash heaps can contain excessive amounts of carbon, nitrogen, and sulfur. The policy and enforcement ramifications affect the poorest coal regions, where some straight pipes still exist and investment in both sewage treatment and storm-water runoff tends to be inadequate. When pollution typical of poor sanitary practices by coal mine operations is found, the polluted water is invariably analyzed for the presence of fecal coliforms as well. When fecal coliforms are found, straight pipes provide an alternative and regionally preferable explanation, despite the presence of massive amounts of organic-range pollutants from fossil fuel extraction, especially coal. This alternative explanation is not necessarily based on science.

Humans are not the only species that defecates or that harbors fecal coliforms. Microbes are fully capable of using carbon and nitrogen and sulfur from multiple sources, and there is no reason to believe that fecal coliforms come from household sewage rather than industrial sources of elements that are essential to bacterial growth. But that is exactly what official reports and regional regulatory agencies routinely conclude.[28]

Fortunately, ongoing commitments of time and resources can partially remediate polluted streams. Perpetual applications of lime have resurrected "dead" streams throughout Appalachia, reversing the effects of acidic mine drainage and creating suitable habitats for even susceptible species, such as native brook trout. These applications reverse pH problems but do not necessarily remove all excess minerals from coal-related activities. Many fishing streams in the coal-burning areas of Appalachia have mercury-based fish consumption warnings, and many residents face potentially high levels of undesirable minerals in potable water. One hopeful development is research aimed at turning coal waste into a resource. Coal-polluted water contains rare earth elements needed in the microelectronic and optics industries. These elements are currently purchased from international suppliers, making the US economy dependent on others for the creation of many highly technical products. Success is uncertain. Determining whether the same process could also improve Appalachian water supplies is a key part of the research effort and of great regional interest.[29]

A recent nationally publicized water crisis in Appalachia illustrates several problems and consequences of misplaced priorities. In 2014 a spill of around 7,500 gallons of a chemical mixture containing primarily 4-methlycyclohexanemethanol (MCHM) effectively shut down the water supply of 380,000 customers in West Virginia's Kanawha Valley for days to weeks. Two million consumers farther downstream experienced less substantial disruptions. Liquid MCHM mixtures are used to clean coal and are stored in bulk quantities. A postincident analysis revealed that state environmental officials were aware that the large containment vessel had been leaking and was past due for replacement. Nevertheless, site inspections were rare, and facility upgrades were not required. There was no automated means of leak detection; the spill was traced to its source by odor. The utility's carbon-filtration systems were not built for industrial-scale events, so water intake had to be shut off. Consumers' water service was resumed five to ten days after the event in different parts of the distribution system. Area businesses closed due to lack of water, creating tremendous losses associated with the foreseeable (but unforeseen) catastrophe. Consumers' problems persisted long after the restoration of water services because water heaters were contaminated and required extensive flushing before the noxious MCHM odor dissipated. It could have been far worse—it could have been a more hazardous chemical. Nevertheless, emergency room and physician visits rose, with patients reporting a variety of signs and symptoms. Post hoc analyses pointed out the difficulty of responding when information about the offending chemicals was not available, toxicity testing by the manufacturer was incomplete, and responses by the relevant agencies were not the subject of advance planning. Efforts to evaluate potential long-term risks or to plan for alternative sources of water when crises occur remain inconsistent in the region.[30]

Receiving far less publicity are the perpetual problems of Appalachian residents who live with poor-quality water on a daily basis, notably in eastern Kentucky and southern West Virginia. Tap water can be "muddy" for days, and boil-water advisories recur frequently. Affected communities generally have aging water infrastructure, sometimes built as part of the original coal camp, and they have few assets for upgrades because the mines causing the pollution are no longer operating. However, new mines, including nearby mountaintop mining, can contribute to the problem. Fixing these problems generally becomes a long-delayed responsibility of all taxpayers in the state, an ongoing legacy of externally shifted industrial costs.

Worker Health

Appalachia has some thoughtful employers that provide sustainable employment opportunities. Some parts of Appalachia lead the nation in highly technical industrial development, occupational health, employer supports for employees' creative living, and environmental stewardship. Overall, however, the history of employment in Appalachia has been, and remains, one of difficulty. For decades, job loss and population stagnation followed in the wake of unsustainable business practices. Diminished worker protection and specific health problems have persisted over decades. Appalachia is the historical home of labor strife and mine wars, including martial law and the deployment of US troops to end armed coal miners' insurrection against armed mercenaries hired by mine owners. The mine wars ended, but economic despair and poor worker health persist in coal country.

The original coal barons created private coal camps, or coal towns, in remote areas. They envisioned creating a stable labor force without incurring the costs or delays associated with the usual organic growth of citizen services. Owners later sold the taxable surface real estate (often to the workers) while maintaining control of the underground mineral rights and the company store.

Just as the coal town was characterized by shortcuts that overlooked normal infrastructure, Appalachian coal country has consistently shortchanged worker health for increasingly implausible promises of long-term employment: the next worker sacrifice is the one that will lead to regional prosperity and job security. Appalachian mineral extraction has created great wealth, but that wealth seldom stays where the workforce lives. The extraction industry is characterized by hidden subsidization of employers, diminished long-term labor opportunities, contingent employment that avoids benefits, reemergence of preventable threats to worker health, and shifting of the costs of industrial illness to regional and national taxpayers.

Coal mining is inherently dangerous. Substantial investment in engineering can reduce the danger of fatal gas exposure, dust and gas explosions, acute traumatic injury from equipment or rockfall, and numerous chronic hazards, including inhaled dust and repetitive trauma from nonergonomic job duties. A single explosion in Monongah, West Virginia, in 1907 took the lives of more than 350 workers, including children. It received more publicity than many other mine disasters of the era, and it led to the creation of the US Bureau of Mines. However, it did not result in the actual reform of mine safety regulations, in contrast to the near-contemporaneous and equally tragic Triangle Shirtwaist fire in New York City in 1911 (death toll 146). The number who died at Monongah is only an estimate, reflecting the careless labor practices in Appalachian coal towns at the time.

Comparison to low- and middle-income countries also illustrates workplace progress. Miners elsewhere in the world experience far more frequent disasters and higher morbidity and mortality rates than those in the United States. There are similar but less marked differences in small versus large, better-organized US mines; these outcomes are generally understood to illustrate that engineering, training, and the use of personal protective equipment can decrease the danger of coal mining. Technological advances in mine ventilation, gas detection, and dust suppression; roof bolting to suppress rockfalls; the use of safer tools; and the wearing of air filtration equipment have all contributed to a century of progress. Yet there are reasons for concern. The economic marginalization of coal by more competitive alternative fuels exerts pressure to cut labor costs, including the costs of worker safety, especially in smaller Appalachian mines. Mine operators seeking to make a profit from the increasingly marginal, narrow coal seams that remain can cut costs by employing a smaller workforce with longer working hours and by hiring independent contractors rather than employees. The contract workforce adds downward pressure on bids and results in less training, safety compliance, and expertise. Narrower seams mean more dust per ton of extracted coal in underground mines, favoring environmentally destructive surface mining for both safety and cost reasons. Longer hours spent in the remaining underground mines can lead to more dust exposure and possibly a diminished protective effect of respirators, given that the correct use of tight-fitting respirators is very uncomfortable over long shifts. Although there has been substantial technological progress in the century since the largest mine disasters occurred, those changes represent only partial success. Ongoing reliance on hard-to-wear personal protective equipment illustrates that more progress is needed.[31]

Recent mine disasters are rooted in regulatory failure. After twelve miners died in explosions in Sago, West Virginia, in 2006, labor representatives noted that small regulatory fines had not altered problematic business practices. Twenty-nine died in the Upper Big Branch Mine in 2010. The Mine Safety and Health Administration (MSHA) had expressed ongoing concerns about that mine operation, and employees described hazardous practices after the disaster. Less visible to the public is the complicity of elected officials who mourn publicly at funerals but exert behind-the-scenes pressure on regulatory and research agencies to relax expensive engineering practices or abrogate fines for violations. A politically dominant industry can quietly but effectively characterize protective and preventive measures as "burdensome" to job preservation before a disaster happens. Rebalancing occurs after a tragedy, but it is often short-lived, as our attention on worker health and disaster planning is focused elsewhere.

Appalachia is the site of America's largest occupational disease disaster. Pneumoconiosis is a lung disease caused by the habitual inhalation of irritants. Black lung and silicosis are types of pneumoconiosis affecting coal miners and some other occupations. Coal dust is more dangerous when it contains crystalline silica. In addition to underground coal mining, rock grinding, cutting, and polishing; surface drilling; and sandblasting can cause silicosis. The disease can be rapidly and inevitably progressive, robbing young workers of breath and health. Based on engineering and personal protective technologies, silicosis should have become a historical footnote. Instead, we have somehow managed to turn back the clock.[32]

To fully understand the danger posed by silicosis, consider this example: The Gauley River in West Virginia is currently cherished for its world-class rapids, white-water rafting excursions, and breathtaking scenery. Nearly a century ago, in the 1930s, an estimated 5,000 short-term workers dug a three-mile-long tunnel through a mountain to replace a bend in the river with a more direct, steeper gradient to supply hydroelectric power to a new metals industry. The mountain's interior was composed largely of crystalline silica, which is valuable for certain specialty metal applications. It is disputed whether the doctors and supervising engineers employed by Union Carbide, the tunnel owner, were aware of the health threat posed by crystalline silica, even though cases of silicosis had already been reported. There is some inferential evidence that they knew. For instance, African American employees were preferentially given interior tunnel jobs, where exposure to silica was more concentrated. Shifts lasted ten to fifteen hours, and tunnel drilling was done "dry," without the use of spray or mist wetting that had been deployed to suppress dust in coal mines. Archive photographs show the underground workers without any kind of respiratory protection or wearing only improvised cloth bandanas. Letters and personnel data suggest that many workers lasted less than six months before the onset of debilitating illness. The US National Park Service and local volunteers have located and marked some of the previously unmarked graves of the estimated 794 men who did not survive long enough to return home. The full toll was higher, of course. A beautiful overlook on Hawk's Nest Mountain above the tunnel contains a memorial. The episode was the subject of a novel and a more recent scholarly work, but because it is an Appalachian story, it is seldom discussed except by public health personnel, social scientists, and residents of coal country. National Public Radio's Adelina Lancianese recently uncovered the company's historic reaction to this tragedy. In response to a congressional inquiry, one company official denied responsibility, stating, "we know of no cases of silicosis contracted on this job." The tunnel still provides hydroelectric power today.[33]

With modern technology, black lung and silicosis were in steep decline by the 1990s, but they are no longer in decline, at least not in eastern Kentucky, southwestern Virginia, or southern West Virginia. Current prevalence levels have not been seen since 1985, and many younger workers are affected. New cases will surely emerge based on recent exposures.[34]

What happened? We will never know all the answers, but we do know that this tragedy is the result of a declining resource combined with insufficient protection. Because the best coal seams have been mined out, access to thinner coal seams requires the removal of greater amounts of "overburden" rock using more efficient drilling techniques. This creates much more coal dust. Longer workdays, part of the strategy to cut costs, increase the amount of dust inhaled each day. Union leaders are obviously correct in their assessment that dust concentrations in ambient air are too high, and the Department of Labor's inspector general is clearly correct in concluding that fines for unsafe practices are not achieving safe working conditions and may instead be seen by mine operators as merely a cost of doing business. These conclusions can be verified by any honest doctor looking at a radiograph. But there is insufficient discussion of how best to tackle the problem of disease caused by unsustainable practices and the inadequacy of benefits to deal with these and other mining-related disabilities. The return of this preventable disease is emblematic of the prioritization of job creation over worker protection. By the time medical imaging confirms the presence of lung injury, the process can be relatively far advanced. Today, lung transplantation can save some lives, but at tremendous financial cost and with diminished health in those who survive.[35]

It is too soon to say whether there will be cases of silicosis in the shale gas industry and its sand suppliers. However, we do know from news and government reports (including one in 2008 by the House Committee on Education and Labor) that the natural gas industry lacks transparency on issues of worker health. It has a high mortality rate (which is almost always reported) but an exceptionally low rate of nonfatal injury. The logical explanation for this discrepancy is injury underreporting. This outcome is abetted by a playbook that is already familiar from the coal industry: aggressive use of bid contractors rather than employees, fewer benefits, and injury underreporting.[36]

The economic politics of injury reporting in different industrial categories and across different regions of the country is a big issue. There are many long-term consequences. For hazardous trades, in which injured workers are seldom employed until retirement age, Social Security disability becomes a national means of subsidizing industries that do not fully fund the burden of the trauma they cause. Compared with the rest of the country, the Social Security disability burden is greater in Appalachia in general and in coal country in particular. There is more than one reason for this disparity, and difficult working conditions are certainly a factor. Beyond that, employers' ability to defund negotiated benefits—including defined pensions—while winking in and out of corporate existence with equipment ownership and mineral rights intact, puts a tremendous burden on taxpayers to support mining costs through the replacement of lost pension benefits. This problem comes before federal lawmakers intermittently. The winners have managed to thrive economically while avoiding liability. The biggest losers are workers denied their pensions. Taxpayers are in the middle, generally unaware that they are subsidizing industry practices that cause human health problems.[37]

Assessment

Appalachia is blessed with natural beauty, a temperate climate, and abundant water and mineral resources; yet large parts of the region have failed to thrive. This is sometimes called a "resource curse." Imprudent environmental planning contributes to economic failure and consistently poor health indicators across Appalachia. The certain knowledge that air pollution, water pollution, and the absence of appropriate infrastructure cause disease is somehow forgotten or challenged when Appalachian workers or residents are threatened. The policy trade-off is routinely framed as a need for jobs, a century-long argument coupled with a promise that has never materialized. Quite simply, policy makers should be asking why investors would be interested in a despoiled landscape with inadequate infrastructure and an unhealthy disease burden.

Geography, including the challenge of mountainous terrain, is important. However, geography alone cannot explain the failures outlined above. Vermont, with a similar topography and equally rural workforce, is consistently among national leaders in health indicators. The median family income in Vermont ($74,426, close to the US average) is significantly higher than the median family income in Appalachia ($60,356) and much higher than the median income in coal country (around $34,000). This is the case even though Vermont has a more challenging climate and a far smaller pool of extractable mineral resources.[38]

Part of the explanation can be found in the decision-maker culture of Appalachia, perpetuating what has been called a century-long failed experiment. Regional utilities' slow pace toward more diverse and less expensive sources of energy puts the region in a less competitive position. Recent tax breaks to encourage the expansion of unviable coal-burning facilities provide a thought-provoking commentary on the long-term economic and environmental impacts of hidden subsidies to the coal industry. Local landowners who have suffered economic losses from activities related to underground extraction have good reason to believe that state regulatory agencies are heavily influenced by the industries they are supposed to regulate. The legal history of the split estate contributes to economic losses on the surface, where people live, and law and policy often favor the owners of the mineral rights below. Recent federal investigations found that state agencies were not collecting required water samples of mine runoff, meaning that pollution problems went undetected. West Virginia agencies also permitted mine operators to apply "substitutes for topsoil" during the reclamation of huge surface mines. The budget for monitoring these massive industrial operations was only $95,000 per year.[39]

A particular problem in Appalachia is the consistent failure of the 1977 Surface Mining Control and Reclamation Act (SMCRA) to address the environmental degradation of surface mining. Officially reclaimed mines need not have adequate soil and timber ground cover to make the land fit for habitation or farming. Springs and perennial streams are permanently buried under fill, and to the degree that water escapes, high concentrations of undesirable minerals are common. The mines operate in human time; time frames for abating their vast historical and ongoing pollution are much longer. The SMCRA's failure to protect Appalachian stream quality and adjacent homeowner property is attributable to inadequate funding, exacerbated by "industry-captive" state agencies.[40]

Geologic and economic assessments predicted the precarious and declining position of Appalachian coal more than three decades ago and called for the diversification of power generation and economic activity. That prediction was based on science, and we now know that it was correct. In coal country, the prediction was ignored, and a "war on coal" narrative was substituted. The region's economic underperformance remains, and worker and environmental needs have been ignored, yet the narrative is still potent, and the policy decisions persist.[41]

Further, the rapid creation of new natural gas wells and pipelines illustrates how poor regional planning combines with regulatory capture to achieve losses where the more reasoned development of infrastructure might lead to permanent gains. Regulatory and public utility agencies have consistently favored the unfettered development of gas wells, followed by parallel pipeline development to export the increasing amounts of gas available. Along the way, homeowner safety and economic concerns have been mostly ignored, and numerous problems in public wildlands—including stream degradation from erosion and silting—have been overlooked. Multiple utility pipelines have become "necessary" because of an unnecessary natural gas glut. These utilities are seeking markets outside of Appalachia and are even looking for international clients, but the cost is borne by regional ratepayers.

So far, courts (rather than regulatory agencies) have provided some balance to environmentally problematic developments, occasionally slowing the pace of extraction so that it can proceed more thoughtfully. Even so, such decisions are hard fought and rare. Exhausting a finite mineral resource as quickly as possible is unlikely to foster major regional development for value-added products that support long-term employment. One can only hope that economically valuable gas will remain once coherent approaches to planning are implemented.[42]

It is reasonable to expect that policy makers in a poor region will favor development. It is less clear why poor decisions with long-term costs are so common. Favoring development should not mean that foreseeable consequences are ignored—a lesson too seldom learned. Developers are routinely permitted to build without shouldering the costs of water delivery, secondary road development and maintenance, sewage transport and treatment, worker health and benefits, and water runoff solutions. Consequences devolve to surface landowners, taxpayers, and utility ratepayers—groups that do not have means to pay, nor the ability to refuse to pay.

Options that are less environmentally destructive are not always considered. From an environmental science perspective, policy makers may not recognize that they have options or even that they are making decisions when new projects do not include sufficient infrastructure to support sustainable development or land reclamation. Nor is the problem limited to major industries. New housing developments are created under similar circumstances, without plans for dealing with storm water, vehicular traffic, or other needs of the built environment. The ongoing Appalachian disappointment in the built environment is partially about the absence of vision and planning, based on the belief that environmental sacrifices are sustainable and necessary. The outcomes have been the opposite of the intention.

Appalachia's lagging economic growth, poor job opportunities, and intermittently despoiled environment are often used to illustrate the concept of a "resource curse." Regions blessed with mineral resources often experience marginal economies. Appalachia's reality is more complex and therefore far more optimistic. Decisions that rely on instant fixes—"if only" solutions—can be avoided. Decisions that anticipate and account for cost shifting, environmental impacts, and preservation, and decisions that respect human health more consistently, can build sustainable economic development. It is not an abstract thought. There are real-life examples of combined economic and environmental success. Asheville and Boone, North Carolina; Bath, New York; Greenville, South Carolina; and Johnson City, Tennessee, have implemented differently scaled, regionally strong approaches to economic stability. Success can be achieved in regions that have not always had that advantage. Differences in wealth between urban and rural economies will always be present. But it is not inevitable that Appalachia will continue to lag behind other regions in health and economic indicators. The turnaround will not be fast. In fact, the last century, with its perceived need for haste, is at the core of the problem. The turnaround will start when the leadership narrative advances from wishful thinking to sound, realistic planning.

Notes

1. Gopal K. Singh et al., "Social Determinants of Health in the United States: Addressing Major Health Inequality Trends for the Nation, 1935-2016," *International Journal of Maternal and Child Health and AIDS* 6, no. 2 (2017): 139-64; "Maps by Topic: Poverty," ARC, 2020, https://www.arc.gov/research/MapsofAppalachia.asp?F_CATEGORY_ID=6; Kelvin Pollard and Linda A. Jacobsen, *The Appalachian Region: A Data Overview from the 2013-2017 Appalachian Community Survey Chartbook* (Washington, DC: ARC, 2019), https://www.arc.gov/assets/research_reports/DataOverviewfrom2013to2017ACS.pdf.

2. Yuka Makino, Sara Manuelli, and Lindsey Hook, "Accelerating the Movement for Mountain Peoples and Policies," *Science* 365, no. 6458 (2019): 1084-86.

3. Ronald L. Lewis, "Deforestation," in *The West Virginia Encyclopedia,* West Virginia Humanities Council, September 19, 2013, https://www.wvencyclopedia.org/articles/1867.

4. Mark Bushnell, "Then Again: When the Green Mountains Were Not so Green," VTDigger, July 15, 2018, https://vtdigger.org/2018/07/15/green-mountains-not-green/.

5. Abee L. Boyles et al., "Systematic Review of Community Health Impacts of Mountaintop Removal Mining," *Environment International* 107 (2017): 163–72; James Bruggers, "Appalachia's Strip-Mined Mountains Face a Growing Climate Risk: Flooding," *Inside Climate News*, November 21, 2019, https://insideclimatenews.org/news/21112019/appalachia-mountains-flood-risk-climate-change-coal-mining-west-virginia-extreme-rainfall-runoff-analysis?fbclid=IwAR3u9RfEOZ7DNQy-lzDRAt0i_IZ2jTW6rucbamL-dijyNqYB-VEp0iKU_B0; Caitlyn Greene and Patrick Charles McGinley, "Yielding to the Necessities of a Great Public Industry: Denial and Concealment of the Harmful Health Effects of Coal Mining," *William & Mary Environmental Law and Policy Review* 43, no. 3 (2019): 689–757.

6. Jeff Hughes et al., *Drinking Water and Wastewater Infrastructure in Appalachia: An Analysis of Capital Funding and Funding Gaps* (Chapel Hill, NC: UNC Environmental Finance Center and ARC, 2005), https://efc.sog.unc.edu/sites/default/files/ARC_FullReport_WithAppendix.pdf.

7. A. R. Brandt et al., "Energy and Environment: Methane Leaks from North American Natural Gas Systems," *Science* 343, no. 6172 (2014): 733–35; Daniel Zavala-Araiza et al., "Reconciling Divergent Estimates of Oil and Gas Methane Emissions," *Proceedings of the National Academy of Sciences of the United States of America* 112, no. 51 (2015): 15597–602; Ramón A. Alvarez et al., "Assessment of Methane Emissions from the U.S. Oil and Gas Supply Chain," *Science* 361, no. 6398 (2018): 186–88; Philip J. Landrigan, Howard Frumkin, and Brita E. Lundberg, "The False Promise of Natural Gas," *New England Journal of Medicine* 382, no. 2 (2020): 104–7; Benjamin Hmiel et al., "Preindustrial (14)CH4 Indicates Greater Anthropogenic Fossil CH4 Emissions," *Nature* 578, no. 7795 (2020): 409–12; Sudhanshu Pandey et al., "Satellite Observations Reveal Extreme Methane Leakage from a Natural Gas Well Blowout," *Proceedings of the National Academy of Sciences of the United States of America* 116, no. 52 (2019): 26376–81.

8. West Virginia Coal Association, "47th Annual Mining Symposium Agenda: Coal Tax Policy," 2020, https://www.wvcoal.com/resources/coal-tax-policy.

9. Laurence Hammack, "Mountain Valley Agrees to Pay $266,000 for Pollution Problems in W.VA," *Roanoke (VA) Times*, May 14, 2019, https://www.roanoke.com/business/mountain-valley-agrees-to-pay-for-pollution-problems-in-w/article_ced1721a-7fc7-5c0b-91f5-b1c5b0a10efb.html.

10. Timothy Fitzgerald, "Understanding Mineral Rights," Montana State University Extension, January 2017, https://store.msuextension.org/publications/AgandNaturalResources/MT201207AG.pdf.

11. Anya Litvak, "CNX Gas Co. and State Regulators Strike Deal over Abandoned Wells," *Pittsburgh Post-Gazette*, October 11, 2019, https://www.post-gazette.com/business/powersource/2019/10/11/CNX-DEP-deal-abandoned-coal-bed-methane-natural-gas-wells-greene-allegheny-washington-westmoreland/stories/201910110146.

12. Craig Howley, *The Rural School Bus Ride in Five States: A Report to the Rural School and Community Trust* (Athens, OH: ERIC Clearinghouse on Rural Education and Small Schools, 2001), http://www.ruraledu.org/user_uploads/Rural_School_Bus_Ride.pdf; Lorna Jimerson, *Slow Motion: Traveling by School Bus in Consolidated Districts in West Virginia* (Arlington, VA: Rural School and Community Trust, 2007), https://files.eric.ed.gov

/fulltext/ED499440.pdf; Motao Zhu et al., "Appalachian versus Non-Appalachian U.S. Traffic Fatalities, 2008–2010," *Annals of Epidemiology* 23, no. 6 (2013): 377–80; James E. Stevenson, Carl Spurlock, and Michele Nypaver, "Factors Associated with the Higher Traumatic Death Rate among Rural Children," *Annals of Emergency Medicine* 27, no. 5 (1996): 625–32; Toni Marie Rudisill et al., "Differences between Occupational and Non-Occupational-Related Motor Vehicle Collisions in West Virginia: A Cross-Sectional and Spatial Analysis," *PLoS One* 14, no. 12 (2019): e0227388.

13. Adam Hege, Richard W. Christiana, Rebecca Battista, and Hannah Parkhurst, "Active Living in Rural Appalachia: Using the Rural Active Living Assessment (RALA) Tools to Explore Environmental Barriers," *Preventive Medicine Reports* 8 (2017): 261–66; Kate Beatty et al., *Creating a Culture of Health in Appalachia: Disparities and Bright Spots* (Princeton, NJ: RWJF, 2019), https://www.arc.gov/assets/research_reports /HealthDisparitiesRelatedtoObesityinAppalachiaApr2019.pdf.

14. Rails to Trails Conservancy, "Economic Benefits of Trails and Greenways," Trails and Greenways Clearinghouse, October 1, 2003, https://www.railstotrails.org /resourcehandler.ashx?id=4618; Terry Easton, "The Business of Trails: A Compilation of Economic Benefits," American Trails, December 31, 2008, https://www.americantrails.org /resources/the-business-of-trails-a-compilation-of-economic-benefits.

15. World Health Organization, "Global Health Observatory Data Repository: Joint Effects of Air Pollution, Data by Country," May 30, 2018, http://apps.who.int/gho/data /view.main.SDGAIRBOD392v?lang=en.

16. Elizabeth T. Jacobs, Jefferey L. Burgess, and Mark B. Abbott, "The Donora Smog Revisited: 70 Years after the Event that Inspired the Clean Air Act," *American Journal of Public Health* 108, no. S2 (2018): S85–88; Donora Historical Society and Smog Museum, "Steel Mill and 1948 Smog," https://www.sites.google.com/site/donorahistoricalsociety /1948-smog. For those interested in the role of unsung women scientists, there is also a brief note about the role of toxicologist Mary Amdur in characterizing how air pollution harms us; the father of a Hall of Fame baseball player is sometimes included among the late victims. Visitors to the Donora Smog Museum or its website can get the flavor of the newsreels that captured the public's attention and led to Americans' willingness to connect air pollution to health outcomes and invest in improved air quality. See also EPA, *The National Air Monitoring Program: Air Quality and Emissions Trends Annual Report*, vol. 1, EPA-450-I-73-001 (Washington, DC: EPA, 1973), https://www.epa.gov/sites/production /files/2017-11/documents/trends_report_1971_v1.pdf.

17. Douglas W. Dockery et al., "An Association between Air Pollution and Mortality in Six U.S. Cities," *New England Journal of Medicine* 329, no. 24 (1993): 1753–59.

18. Zhuanlan Sun and Demi Zhu, "Exposure to Outdoor Air Pollution and Its Human Health Outcomes: A Scoping Review," *PLoS One* 14, no. 5 (2019): e0216550; Regina Rückerl et al., "Health Effects of Particulate Air Pollution: A Review of Epidemiological Evidence," *Inhalation Toxicology* 23, no. 10 (2011): 555–92; Anna Oudin et al., "Traffic-Related Air Pollution as a Risk Factor for Dementia: No Clear Modifying Effects of APOEe4 in the Betula Cohort," *Journal of Alzheimer's Disease* 71, no. 3 (2019): 733–40; Rob Beelen et al., "Effects of Long-Term Exposure to Air Pollution on Natural-Cause Mortality: An Analysis of 22 European Cohorts within the Multicentre ESCAPE Project," *Lancet* 383, no. 9919 (2014): 785–95; Ole Raaschou-Nielsen et al., "Air Pollution and Lung Cancer Incidence in 17 European Cohorts: Prospective Analyses from the European Study of Cohorts for Air

Pollution Effects (ESCAPE)," *Lancet Oncology* 14, no. 9 (2013): 813–22; C. Arden Pope III, Majid Ezzati, and Douglas W. Dockery, "Fine-Particulate Air Pollution and Life Expectancy in the United States," *New England Journal of Medicine* 360, no. 4 (2009): 376–86.

19. Mark Byrnes, "What Pittsburgh Looked Like When It Decided It Had a Pollution Problem," CityLab, June 5, 2012, https://www.citylab.com/design/2012/06/what-pittsburgh-looked-when-it-decided-it-had-pollution-problem/2185/; American Lung Association, "State of the Air 2019," https://www.lung.org/our-initiatives/healthy-air/sota/; Mick Mulvaney, "Office of Management and Budget (OMB) Bulletin No. 18-04: Revised Delineations of Metropolitan Statistical Areas, and Combined Statistical Areas, and Guidance on Uses of the Delineations of These Areas," 2018, https://www.whitehouse.gov/wp-content/uploads/2018/09/Bulletin-18-04.pdf.

20. Leigh-Anne Krometis et al., "Environmental Health Disparities in the Central Appalachian Region of the United States," *Reviews on Environmental Health* 32, no. 3 (2017): 253–66; Laura Kurth et al., "Atmospheric Particulate Matter in Proximity to Mountaintop Coal Mines: Sources and Potential Environmental and Human Health Impacts," *Environmental Geochemistry and Health* 37, no. 3 (2015): 529–44; Laura M. Kurth, Michael McCawley, Michael Hendryx, and Stephanie Lusk, "Atmospheric Particulate Matter Size Distribution and Concentration in West Virginia Coal Mining and Non-Mining Areas," *Journal of Exposure Science & Environmental Epidemiology* 24, no. 4 (2014): 405–11; A. K. Salm and Michael J. Benson, "Increased Dementia Mortality in West Virginia Counties with Mountaintop Removal Mining?" *International Journal of Environmental Research and Public Health* 16, no. 21 (2019): 4278; Viney P. Aneja et al., "Particulate Matter Pollution in the Coal-Producing Regions of the Appalachian Mountains: Integrated Ground-Based Measurements and Satellite Analysis," *Journal of the Air & Waste Management Association* 67, no. 4 (2017): 421–30; American Lung Association, "State of the Air 2019"; Melissa M. Ahern et al., "The Association between Mountaintop Mining and Birth Defects among Live Births in Central Appalachia, 1996–2003," *Environmental Research* 111, no. 6 (2011): 838–46; Michael Hendryx, "Mortality from Heart, Respiratory, and Kidney Disease in Coal Mining Areas of Appalachia," *International Archives of Occupational and Environmental Health* 82, no. 2 (2009): 243–49.

21. Christopher M. Long, Nicole L. Briggs, and Ifeoluwa A. Bamgbose, "Synthesis and Health-Based Evaluation of Ambient Air Monitoring Data for the Marcellus Shale Region," *Journal of the Air & Waste Management Association* 69, no. 5 (2019): 527–47; Michael A. McCawley, "Does Increased Traffic Flow around Unconventional Resource Development Activities Represent the Major Respiratory Hazard to Neighboring Communities? Knowns and Unknowns," *Current Opinion in Pulmonary Medicine* 23, no. 2 (2017): 161–66; Elise G. Elliott et al., "A Community-Based Evaluation of Proximity to Unconventional Oil and Gas Wells, Drinking Water Contaminants, and Health Symptoms in Ohio," *Environmental Research* 167 (2018): 550–57; Ashley L. Bolden, Kim Schultz, Katherine E. Pelch, and Carol F. Kwiatkowski, "Exploring the Endocrine Activity of Air Pollutants Associated with Unconventional Oil and Gas Extraction," *Environmental Health* 17, no. 1 (2018): 26; Janet Currie, Michael Greenstone, and Katherine Meckel, "Hydraulic Fracturing and Infant Health: New Evidence from Pennsylvania," *Science Advances* 3, no. 12 (2017): e1603021; Joan A. Casey, David A. Savitz, et al., "Unconventional Natural Gas Development and Birth Outcomes in Pennsylvania, USA," *Epidemiology* 27, no. 2 (2016): 163–72; Joan A. Casey, Dana E. Goin, et al., "Unconventional Natural Gas Development and Adverse Birth Outcomes in Pennsylvania: The Potential Mediating Role of Antenatal Anxiety and Depres-

sion," *Environmental Research* 177 (2019): 108598; Aaron W. Tustin et al., "Associations between Unconventional Natural Gas Development and Nasal and Sinus, Migraine Headache, and Fatigue Symptoms in Pennsylvania," *Environmental Health Perspectives* 125, no. 2 (2017): 189–97; John A. Casey et al., "Associations of Unconventional Natural Gas Development with Depression Symptoms and Disordered Sleep in Pennsylvania," *Scientific Reports* 8, no. 1 (2018): 11375.

22. Krometis et al., "Environmental Health Disparities"; Kurth et al., "Atmospheric Particulate Matter in Proximity"; Kurth et al., "Atmospheric Particulate Matter Size"; Aneja et al., "Particulate Matter Pollution"; Bolden et al., "Exploring the Endocrine Activity"; James E. Bennett et al., "Particulate Matter Air Pollution and National and County Life Expectancy Loss in the USA: A Spatiotemporal Analysis," *PLoS Medicine* 16, no. 7 (2019): e1002856.

23. Nathaniel C. Skaggs, "Trout Fishing in the Smokies and the Blue Ridge, 1880–Present: How-to, History, and Habitat" (master's thesis, East Tennessee State University, 2017), https://dc.etsu.edu/cgi/viewcontent.cgi?article=4629&context=etd; Barton D. Clinton and James M. Vose, "Variation in Stream Water Quality in an Urban Headwater Stream in the Southern Appalachians," *Water, Air, and Soil Pollution* 169 (2006): 331–53.

24. *The Buffalo Creek Flood and Disaster: Official Report of the Governor's Ad Hoc Commission of Inquiry* (Charleston: State of West Virginia, 1973), http://www.wvculture.org /HISTORY/disasters/buffcreekgovreport.html.

25. Brian D. Drollette et al., "Elevated Levels of Diesel Range Organic Compounds in Groundwater Near Marcellus Gas Operations Are Derived from Surface Activities," *Proceedings of the National Academy of Sciences of the United States of America* 112, no. 43 (2015): 13184–89.

26. Robert B. Jackson et al., "Increased Stray Gas Abundance in a Subset of Drinking Water Wells Near Marcellus Shale Gas Extraction," *Proceedings of the National Academy of Sciences of the United States of America* 110, no. 28 (2013): 11250–55.

27. Wendee Nicole, "CAFOs and Environmental Justice: The Case of North Carolina," *Environmental Health Perspectives* 121, no. 6 (2013): A182–89.

28. Coal is generally 0.5 to 2.0 percent nitrogen content and 0.4 to 4.0 percent sulfur content, depending on the geology and use.

29. Daniel M. Downey, Christopher R. French, and Michael Odom, "Low Cost Limestone Treatment of Acid Sensitive Trout Streams in Appalachian Waters of Virginia," *Water, Air, and Soil Pollution* 77 (1994): 49–77.

30. A. J. Whelton et al., "Case Study: The Crude MCHM Chemical Spill Investigation and Recovery in West Virginia USA," *Environmental Science, Water Research, and Technology* 3 (2017): 312–32.

31. International Labour Organization, "Mining: A Hazardous Work," March 23, 2015, https://www.ilo.org/global/topics/safety-and-health-at-work/areasofwork/hazardous -work/WCMS_356567/lang-en/index.htm.

32. Eric J. Esswein et al., "Occupational Exposures to Respirable Crystalline Silica during Hydraulic Fracturing," *Journal of Occupational and Environmental Hygiene* 10, no. 7 (2013): 347–56.

33. Adelina Lancianese, "Before Black Lung, the Hawk's Nest Tunnel Disaster Killed Hundreds," National Public Radio, January 20, 2019, https://www.npr.org/2019/01/20 /685821214/before-black-lung-the-hawks-nest-tunnel-disaster-killed-hundreds; National Park Service, "The Hawk's Nest Tunnel Disaster: Summerville, WV," January 22, 2020, https://www.nps.gov/neri/planyourvisit/the-hawks-nest-tunnel-disaster-summersville-wv

.htm; Sheldon Rampton and John Stauber, "Dying for a Living," in *Trust Us, We're Experts: How Industry Manipulates Science and Gambles with Your Future* (New York: Putnam, 2001), 75–98. The Hawk's Nest tunnel disaster is fictionalized in Hubert Skidmore, *Hawk's Nest* (Knoxville: University of Tennessee Press, 2004); for academic coverage of this event, see Jock McCulloch, Geoffrey Tweedale, and Anthony J. Lanza, "Silicosis and the Gauley Bridge 'Nine,'" *Social History of Medicine* 27, no. 1 (2014): 86–103.

34. Robert A. Cohen et al., "Lung Pathology in U.S. Coal Workers with Rapidly Progressive Pneumoconiosis Implicates Silica and Silicates," *American Journal of Respiratory and Critical Care Medicine* 193, no. 6 (2016): 673–80; Noemi B. Hall, David J. Blackey, Cara N. Halldin, and A. Scott Laney, "Current Review of Pneumoconiosis among US Coal Miners," *Current Environmental Health Reports* (2019), https://link.springer.com/article/10.1007%2Fs40572-019-00246-4.

35. David Sparkman, "MSHA Seeks More Info on Silica Black Lung," *EHS Today*, October 8, 2019, https://www.ehstoday.com/msha/msha-seeks-more-info-silica-black-lung.

36. Antonia Juhasz, "Death on the Dakota Access," *Pacific Standard Magazine*, September 12, 2018, https://psmag.com/magazine/death-on-the-dakota-access; Committee on Education and Labor, *Hidden Tragedy: Underreporting of Workplace Injuries and Illnesses* (Washington, DC: US House of Representatives, 2008), 17.

37. John Gettens, Pei-Pei Li, and Alexis D. Henry, "Accounting for Geographic Variation in Social Security Disability Program Participation," *Social Security Bulletin* 78, no. 2 (2018): 29–47, https://www.ssa.gov/policy/docs/ssb/v78n2/v78n2p29.html.

38. Vermont Department of Numbers, "Vermont Household Income," https://www.deptofnumbers.com/income/vermont/; Commonwealth Fund, "2020 Scorecard on State Health System Performance," https://scorecard.commonwealthfund.org/rankings; Pollard and Jacobsen, *Appalachian Region.*

39. Bernard D. Goldstein, "The Importance of Public Health Agency Independence: Marcellus Shale Gas Drilling in Pennsylvania," *American Journal of Public Health* 104, no. 2 (2014): e13–15; Mason Adams, "A 40-Year-Old Federal Law Literally Changed the Appalachian Landscape," West Virginia Public Broadcasting, August 5, 2017, https://www.wvpublic.org/post/40-year-old-federal-law-literally-changed-appalachian-landscape#stream/0; Ken Ward Jr., "WV DEP Lax in Its Mining Oversight, 3-Year Federal Investigation Says," *Charleston (WV) Gazette-Mail*, February 7, 2017, https://www.wvgazettemail.com/news/politics/wv-dep-lax-in-its-mining-oversight-year-federal/article_fd362370-cef1-5998-bf2b-6bb43463137c.html.

40. Surface Mining Control and Reclamation Act of 1977, Pub. L. No. 95-87, https://www.osmre.gov/lrg.shtm; EPA, *The Effects of Mountaintop Mines and Valley Fills on Aquatic Ecosystems of the Central Appalachian Coal Fields*, EPA600/R-09/138F (Washington, DC: EPA, 2011), https://cfpub.epa.gov/si/si_public_record_report.cfm?Lab=NCEA&dirEntryId=225743.

41. Robert C. Milici, "Depletion of Appalachian Coal Reserves—How Soon?" *International Journal of Coal Geology* 44, no. 3–4 (2000): 251–66.

42. Brittany Patterson, "Atlantic Coast Pipeline Developer Stops Construction," West Virginia Public Broadcasting, December 10, 2018, https://www.wvpublic.org/post/atlantic-coast-pipeline-developer-stops-construction#stream/0.

8

Deaths of Despair in Appalachia

MICHAEL MEIT, MEGAN HEFFERNAN, AND ERIN TANENBAUM

Over the past several years, a growing body of research has been compiled on "deaths of despair," a term first used in 2015 by Case and Deaton.[1] Their initial research demonstrated increasing mortality among the middle-aged white population between 1993 and 2013 from three main causes: overdose (from prescription and illicit drug use and alcohol), suicide, and alcoholic liver disease or cirrhosis of the liver. Collectively, these causes are referred to as deaths of despair. The rise in overdose mortality since 1999 has been particularly notable, driven largely by the opioid crisis. The number of overdose deaths involving opioids increased almost sixfold from 1999 to 2018 across the United States. During that same period, the suicide rate increased by 35 percent, and deaths attributed to alcoholic liver disease or cirrhosis increased by 16 percent. Given the similarity between the demographic profile of much of Appalachia and the populations identified by Case and Deaton as being at higher risk for deaths of despair, the NORC Walsh Center for Rural Health Analysis, with funding from the Appalachian Regional Commission (ARC), first explored deaths of despair in the region using data from 1999 to 2015.[2] NORC then partnered with the East Tennessee State University Center for Rural Health Research (ETSU) to update this study, extending the analysis to include data through 2018.[3]

The NORC/ETSU study aimed to detect differences in mortality rates from deaths of despair between the Appalachian region and the non-Appalachian United States. In addition, it explored differences by age groups and gender. Appalachian rates were further analyzed by Appalachian subregion, county economic status, and levels of rurality. Levels of rurality were based on ARC designations, which are a simplification of the US Department of Agriculture's Economic Research Service (ERS) 2013 urban influence codes (UICs). Additionally, counties were analyzed on their ARC economic classification (described in more detail in chapter 4), based on an index of three economic indicators: three-year unemployment rate, per capita market income, and poverty rate. Mortality data were drawn from the National Vital Statistics System (NVSS) multiple cause of death database compiled by the National Center for Health Statistics (NCHS).

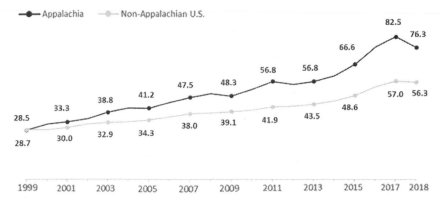

Figure 8.1. Annual mortality rates attributable to deaths of despair, ages 15–64 years, by region (1999–2018). (*Source:* CDC and NCHS, "CDC Wonder," 2020, http://wonder.cdc.gov/mcd-icd10.html)

Rates are age-adjusted and are presented as deaths per 100,000 population.

In all years except 1999, Appalachian and non-Appalachian US rates are significantly different ($p \le 0.05$).

Trends in Mortality Due to Deaths of Despair

From the late 1990s to 2017, the mortality rate due to deaths of despair increased across the United States, and the gap widened between the Appalachian region and the rest of the nation. In 2018 both the Appalachian region and the non-Appalachian United States experienced a decline in mortality due to deaths of despair. As shown in figure 8.1, the mortality rates attributable to deaths of despair in Appalachia and in the non-Appalachian United States were nearly identical in 1999. By 2009, the mortality rate in the Appalachian region was 24 percent higher than in the non-Appalachian United States; by 2017, this difference had increased to 45 percent. Between 2009 and 2017, the mortality rate attributable to deaths of despair in Appalachia nearly tripled. Between 2017 and 2018, the mortality rate declined by 7.5 percent in the Appalachian region, narrowing the gap between Appalachia and the rest of the nation.

As shown in figure 8.2, the mortality rate in 2018 for the combined deaths of despair among those aged fifteen to sixty-four was 76.3 deaths per 100,000 population in Appalachian counties, compared with 56.3 deaths per 100,000 population in non-Appalachian counties. Among the three causes of death (overdose, suicide, and liver disease), the disparity between Appalachia and the non-Appalachian United States was greatest for overdose deaths. In 2018

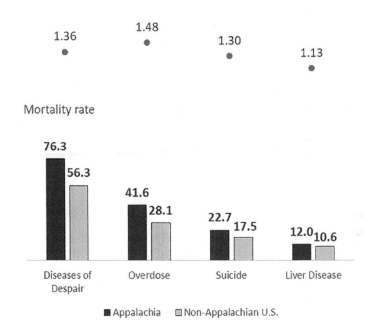

Figure 8.2. Mortality rates attributable to deaths of despair, ages 15–64 years, by disease and region (2018). (*Source:* CDC and NCHS, "CDC Wonder," 2020, http://wonder.cdc.gov/mcd-icd10.html)

Rates are age-adjusted and are presented as deaths per 100,000 population.

For all diseases, Appalachian and non-Appalachian US rates are significantly different ($p \leq 0.05$).

the overdose mortality rate was 48 percent higher in Appalachia than in the non-Appalachian United States (41.6 versus 28.1 deaths per 100,000 population). The suicide mortality rate was 30 percent higher in Appalachia, and the liver disease mortality rate was 13 percent higher. Notably, the proportion of deaths attributable to suicide rose from 20 percent higher in Appalachia in 2015 to 30 percent higher in 2017. This jump represented a 50 percent increase compared with the rest of the United States in just a two-year period.

Disparities within Appalachia

As a whole, the 420-county Appalachian region experiences disparities with the rest of the United States related to deaths of despair. However, disparities

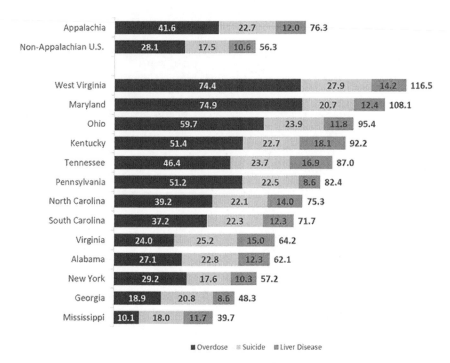

Figure 8.3. Mortality rates attributable to deaths of despair, ages 15–64 years, by region, state, and disease (2018). (*Source:* CDC and NCHS, "CDC Wonder," 2020, http://wonder.cdc.gov/mcd-icd10.html)

Rates are age-adjusted and are presented as deaths per 100,000 population.

For states within Appalachia, only the mortality rate for Appalachian counties is shown.

also exist *within* Appalachia, based on subregion, state, economic status, and rurality.

Exploring mortality rates by state reveals that certain states within Appalachia disproportionately experience deaths of despair and their impact. Figure 8.3 shows the mortality rate for each of the three deaths of despair by state; only the mortality rate for the Appalachian portion of each state is shown. For all deaths of despair, West Virginia and Appalachian Maryland had the highest overall mortality rate, at 116.5 and 108.1 deaths per 100,000 population, respectively. The Appalachian portions of Mississippi, Georgia, and New York had the lowest combined mortality rates from deaths of despair. In Appalachian Maryland, West Virginia, Appalachian Ohio, and Appalachian Pennsylvania, at least 60 percent of these deaths were due to overdose.

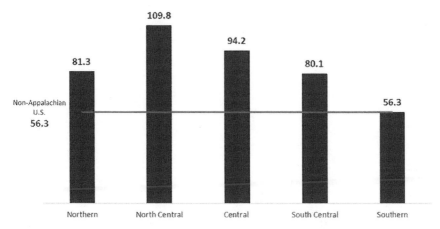

Figure 8.4. Mortality rates attributable to deaths of despair, ages 15–64 years, by subregion (2018). (*Source:* CDC and NCHS, "CDC Wonder," 2020, http://wonder.cdc.gov/mcd-icd10.html)

Rates are age-adjusted and are presented as deaths per 100,000 population.

Within Appalachian subregions, deaths of despair were most common in Central and North Central Appalachia (figure 8.4). In 2018 North Central Appalachia had a mortality rate from deaths of despair of 109.8 deaths per 100,000 population, which was 17 percent higher than the rate in Central Appalachia, 35 percent higher than in Northern Appalachia, 37 percent higher than in South Central Appalachia, and 95 percent higher than in Southern Appalachia. Southern Appalachia had the lowest mortality rate from deaths of despair, at 56.3 deaths per 100,000 population, equal to the mortality rate in the non-Appalachian United States.

This picture is complicated by gender-based disparities. Figure 8.5 shows mortality rates from deaths of despair by gender. Although males had a significantly higher mortality rate than females, the disparity between the Appalachian region and the non-Appalachian United States was greater for females. Among males, the mortality rate for deaths of despair was 31 percent higher in Appalachia than in the non-Appalachian United States. For females, the Appalachian mortality rate was 46 percent higher.

Figure 8.6 shows the mortality rate for each death of despair, comparing "distressed" counties with those in other categories ("at risk," "transitional," "competitive," and "attainment") and therefore considered "nondistressed." While overdose deaths were most common among the three deaths of despair,

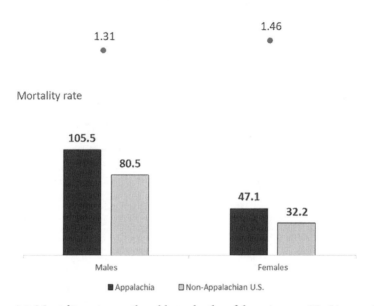

Figure 8.5. Mortality rates attributable to deaths of despair, ages 15–64 years, by gender and region (2018). (*Source:* CDC and NCHS, "CDC Wonder," 2020, http://wonder.cdc.gov/mcd-icd10.html)

Rates are age-adjusted and are presented as deaths per 100,000 population.

For both genders, Appalachian and non-Appalachian US rates are significantly different ($p \leq 0.05$).

the disparity between distressed and nondistressed counties was greatest for liver disease (57 percent higher in distressed counties).

Patterns also appear based on county economic status and rurality (figure 8.7). In nonmetropolitan (nonmetro) counties, the suicide rate was 17 percent higher than in metropolitan (metro) counties, and the mortality rate for liver disease was 23 percent higher. The overdose rate, however, was 13 percent lower in nonmetro than in metro counties. Between the mid-2000s and 2011, the nonmetro counties in Appalachia experienced higher overdose mortality rates than metro counties; this was followed by a narrowing of the disparity between 2011 and 2013, as the overdose mortality rate in nonmetro counties declined. Metro counties experienced a dramatic increase in overdose deaths between 2014 and 2017, which led to higher rates of overdose mortality in metro counties than in nonmetro counties. Then, between 2017 and 2018, the overdose mortality declined by 17 percent in metro Appalachian counties,

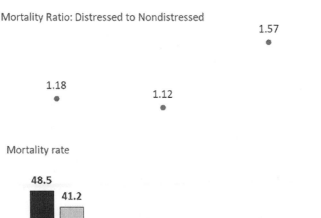

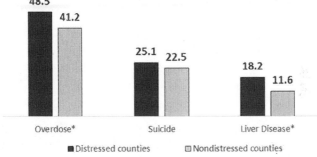

Figure 8.6. Mortality rates attributable to deaths of despair, ages 15–64 years, by disease and county economic status (2018). (*Source:* CDC and NCHS, "CDC Wonder," 2020, http://wonder.cdc.gov/mcd-icd10.html)

Rates are age-adjusted and are presented as deaths per 100,000 population.

*Rates for distressed and nondistressed counties are significantly different ($p \leq 0.05$).

compared with a 6 percent decline in nonmetro counties. These trends are likely attributable to differences in opioid use patterns between metro and nonmetro counties, such as prescription versus injection drug use and their associated lethality.

Overdose Deaths in Appalachia

In 2008 research conducted by NORC and ETSU found disparities in the Appalachian region in terms of substance use and mental health disorders. Specifically, this study observed a growing opioid problem in the region. Other findings include a higher prevalence of mental health disorders, including serious psychological distress and major depressive disorder.[4] The opioid epidemic is discussed in more detail in the next chapter, but the data presented here provide an important preface to that analysis, highlighting drug abuse patterns in Appalachian counties versus the non-Appalachian United States.

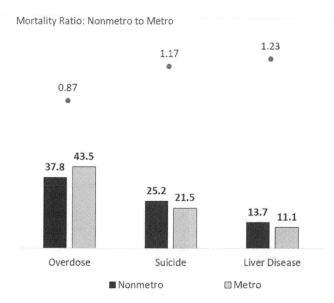

Figure 8.7. Mortality rates attributable to deaths of despair, ages 15–64 years, by disease and rurality (2018). (*Source:* CDC and NCHS, "CDC Wonder," 2020, http://wonder.cdc.gov/mcd-icd10.html)

Rates are age-adjusted and are presented as deaths per 100,000 population.

For all diseases, rates for nonmetro and metro counties are significantly different ($p \leq 0.05$).

More recent analyses of Appalachian data show similar trends related to overdose mortality. Overdose deaths became increasingly common in the decade prior to 2017, largely due to the opioid crisis. In the Appalachian region in 2018, there were 6,483 overdose deaths among those aged fifteen to sixty-four years, and 70 percent of these deaths were caused by opioids (opium, heroin, methadone, other opioids, and synthetic narcotics).

Overdose mortality particularly affects Appalachian adults in their prime working years, between the ages of twenty-five and forty-four (table 8.1). Among males in Appalachia, mortality was highest among those aged twenty-five to thirty-four years (70.9 deaths per 100,000 population) and among those aged thirty-five to forty-four (81.2 deaths per 100,000 population). These age groups also experienced the highest mortality rates in the non-Appalachian United States, although large disparities were observed when comparing Appalachian and non-Appalachian counties. Specifically, the overdose mortality rate was 61 percent higher among males aged thirty-five to forty-four and 49 percent higher among males aged twenty-five to thirty-four in Appalachia than in the non-Appalachian United States. Although the total number of

Table 8.1. Overdose Mortality Rates, Ages 15–64 Years (2018)

Age (Years)	Appalachia	Non-Appalachian US
Male		
15–24	16.2	13.7
25–34	70.9	47.6
35–44	81.2	50.3
45–54	52.7	45.6
55–64	35.8	37.1
Female		
15–24	10.9	5.9
25–34	35.5	18.8
35–44	42.2	21.1
45–54	33.3	21.5
55–64	21.2	17.1

Source: CDC and NCHS, "CDC Wonder," 2020, http://wonder.cdc.gov/mcd-icd10.html.

Note: Mortality rates are presented as deaths per 100,000 population.

overdose deaths was lower among females, the disparity between Appalachia and the non-Appalachian United States was greater for females than for males. Similar to males, females in Appalachia in their prime working years were most affected, with females aged twenty-five to thirty-four experiencing 35.5 overdose deaths per 100,000 population, and those aged thirty-five to forty-four experiencing 42.2 deaths per 100,000 population. The overdose mortality rate for Appalachian females aged twenty-five to thirty-four years was 89 percent higher than the rate in the non-Appalachian United States, and for those aged thirty-five to forty-four, it was double the non-Appalachian rate.

Discussion

These findings document the scale and scope of the challenge in Appalachia, and they highlight the need for additional research on and discussion of effective interventions, policies, and strategies to address these causes of death. In the first two decades of the twenty-first century, deaths from overdose, suicide, and alcoholic liver diseases or cirrhosis increased across the entire United States, but the disparity between Appalachia and the non-Appalachian United States grew considerably. Within Appalachia, the burden is highest in the Central and North Central subregions, where the majority of economically distressed counties are located. Economic development strategies and interventions that address other underlying contributors to deaths of despair—in addition to greater access to treatment and prevention services—may be important considerations in addressing this problem.

The rise in opioid overdose deaths over the past two decades has contributed to the recent increase in deaths of despair, although rising suicide rates in the region are also notable. States with the highest mortality rates from overdose in the Appalachian region are those that have been most significantly impacted by the opioid crisis, as shown by the large percentage of overdose deaths attributed specifically to opioids. When comparing Appalachia and the non-Appalachian United States, the most notable disparities in overdose deaths exist for those aged twenty-five to forty-four years. Working-age adults in Appalachia are considerably more likely to die from an overdose than are similar-aged adults in the rest of the United States. This has significant implications, particularly in terms of economic development.

Finally, it is worth noting that although the most recent data available, from 2018, showed marked declines in overdose mortality, this may not indicate a downward trend. Preliminary data from 2019 have shown increasing rates, and anecdotal information from 2020 indicates that overdose rates may be spiking in association with the COVID-19 pandemic.[5] Similarly, COVID-19 is likely to negatively influence mortality rates from suicide and alcoholic liver disease. It is important to continue tracking deaths of despair in the Appalachian region to assess the long-term impacts of COVID-19 and related factors tied to social isolation, increased joblessness, and limited access to in-person treatment services.

Notes

1. Anne Case and Angus Deaton, "Rising Morbidity and Mortality in Midlife among White Non-Hispanic Americans in the 21st Century," *Proceedings of the National Academy of Sciences of the United States of America* 112, no. 49 (2015): 15078–83.

2. M. Meit, M. Heffernan, E. Tanenbaum, and T. Hoffmann, "Appalachian Diseases of Despair," Appalachian Regional Commission (2017), https://www.arc.gov/wp-content /uploads/2020/06/AppalachianDiseasesofDespairAugust2017.pdf.

3. M. Meit, M. Heffernan, E. Tanenbaum, M. Cherney, and V. Hallman, "Appalachian Diseases of Despair," Appalachian Regional Commission (2020), https://www.arc.gov/wp -content/uploads/2020/11/Appalachian-Diseases-of-Despair-October-2020.pdf.

4. Z. Zhang, A. Infante, M. Meit, and N. English, "An Analysis of Mental Health and Substance Abuse Disparities & Access to Treatment Services in the Appalachian Region," Appalachian Regional Commission (2008), https://www.arc.gov/wp-content/uploads/2020 /06/AnalysisofMentalHealthandSubstanceAbuseDisparities.pdf.

5. F. B. Ahmad, L. M. Rossen, and P. Sutton, "Provisional Drug Overdose Death Counts," National Center for Health Statistics, https://www.cdc.gov/nchs/nvss/vsrr/drug -overdose-data.htm.

9

The Opioid Crisis in Appalachia

Angela Hagaman, Bill Brooks, Stephanie M. Mathis, Kelly E. Moore, and Robert Pack

As of 2017, 1.7 million people in the United States were suffering from a substance use disorder (SUD) related to prescription opioid pain relievers (OPRs), with another 652,000 suffering from a heroin use disorder. Opioids, both prescribed and illicit, were implicated in the early deaths of nearly 400,000 people between 1999 and 2017, which is more than half of all overdose deaths during that period. Presently, more than 130 people in the United States die each day from an opioid overdose, making it the leading cause of injury-related death in the country. Some regions—Appalachia, the mid-Atlantic states, and the rural Northeast—carry a disproportionate burden of opioid use disorder (OUD), and they have been experiencing the negative effects of this crisis for more than a decade (see chapter 8). Current research now demonstrates that approximately 25 percent of counties in the United States have a severe, persistent problem with opioid overdose mortality, with many of those counties clustered in Central Appalachia and the mid-Atlantic states. SUD (and its associated mortality) has been a public health issue for centuries, but never at the magnitude seen today. Appalachian communities in particular have borne this heavy burden due to a confluence of factors outlined in this chapter.[1]

Three Waves of the Opioid Overdose Crisis

Since the early 1990s there have been at least three overlapping waves of opioid overdose deaths in the United States. This trend started with the widespread increase in opioid overdoses fueled by the overprescription of pain-relieving medications (such as Oxycontin) that pharmaceutical companies initially claimed were safe and effective. It was during this period that the prescribing and dispensing of opioids proliferated at a scale previously unknown. The sharp rise in OPR consumption that triggered the current opioid crisis has many drivers, but some have linked it to the pharmaceutical industry's marketing practices. For example, a one-paragraph letter of only 100 words that was published in the *New England Journal of Medicine* in 1980 was subsequently cited as evidence that addiction was rare with long-term opioid therapy, thus beginning the narrative that OPRs were safe. A 1989 study of twenty-eight patients similarly concluded that cancer patients could take prescription opioids for months without becoming addicted. These reports would serve as a cornerstone of the pharmaceutical industry's marketing initiatives launched in the mid-1990s that became known as the "War on Pain." This resulted in hospital accreditation standards that included patient satisfaction scores for pain management, the "pain as the 5th vital sign" campaign, and patient advocacy groups that focused on access to pain medications.[2]

In response to the overwhelming increase in mortality—deemed an epidemic by the Centers for Disease Control and Prevention (CDC)—public health agencies and legislators mobilized to understand the problem and find solutions. Early on, the public's access to vast amounts of OPRs was identified as a major contributing factor to increased mortality, and analyses found that prescribing rates closely paralleled overdose rates. Although much of the prescribing of opioids was done in good faith, a large number of pills were distributed through a profit-first business model that greatly contributed to the number of opioids "in the wild." Prescribing and dispensing data tell the story of a dramatic increase in the prescribing of opioid analgesics over the past ten to fifteen years. Forty-seven million prescriptions for opioid analgesics were written in 2006, and in the last quarter of 2012, prescription volume peaked at 62 million. Pharmaceutical companies sold 76 billion oxycodone and hydrocodone pain pills from 2006 to 2012, according to a database maintained by the Drug Enforcement Administration (DEA).[3]

The marketing of prescription opioids was particularly effective in Appalachia due to high rates of chronic pain, inadequate regulatory oversight, and little public health education about the risk of misuse. Data from the DEA show that the top four states with the most prescription opioids per person are West Virginia, Kentucky, South Carolina, and Tennessee, all of which are located in Appalachia either in whole (West Virginia) or in part. Overdose mortality rates in these states were three times the national average from 2012 to 2016. Thirteen counties had more than eight times the national rate; seven of those thirteen counties were in West Virginia, which led the nation in overdose deaths in 2020. A 2006 review of death records in West Virginia—where more than 34 percent of the population lives in rural communities—found that 93.2 percent of all overdose deaths were among individuals with prescriptions for OPRs. Norton, Virginia, provides another example. From 2006 to 2012, drug companies shipped an average of 306 pain pills per person to this municipality with fewer than 4,000 residents, resulting in an overdose mortality rate eighteen times the national average.[4]

Nationally, the rise in overdose deaths was greatest in nonmetropolitan communities, increasing more than 159 percent between 1999 and 2004. In

Appalachia, 76 percent of the population lives outside of a metropolitan region, and those at greatest risk for fatal and nonfatal overdose during this period were white males between the ages of thirty and thirty-nine years with lower educational attainment, chronic pain, and a history of substance use. Keyes and colleagues have proposed four factors that may explain the differential increase in OPR misuse between rural and urban communities during the first wave of the opioid epidemic. First, as already mentioned, an overall increase in opioid prescriptions led to a surplus of opioids available for diversion and misuse. Second, many young adults migrated from rural areas seeking employment and higher education, leading to a concentration of individuals at high risk for SUD. Third, the highly cohesive family and social networks common in rural areas facilitated the diversion of OPRs across a larger portion of the population. Finally, ongoing and increasing economic hardship in rural communities contributed to social and environmental stressors on the population, increasing the risk of SUD. All these elements converge in Appalachia, specifically in Central Appalachia, where some of the highest rates of overdoses occur nationally.[5]

To counter the overprescribing of OPRs, legislation was enacted. One strategy required physicians and pharmacists to participate in prescription drug monitoring programs (PDMPs), which maintained online records of prescribing and dispensing. The second wave of opioid overdose deaths began as multiple efforts to constrain the supply of prescription opioids proved successful. In 2007 the number of overdose deaths attributable to OPRs in the United States was greater than those associated with heroin and cocaine combined. In 2010 deaths associated with OPRs dropped, and heroin overdose deaths tripled. There is a clear link between these behavioral trends: research indicates that 80 percent of people who use heroin report that they first misused prescription opioids. Analyses of national surveillance data at the time found that individuals reporting past-month heroin use were nineteen times more likely to have a history of nonmedical opioid analgesic use, suggesting that the rise in OPR misuse led directly to an increased demand for heroin. Large demographic shifts were observed in the population of individuals seeking treatment for heroin use during this time, from predominantly nonwhite urban groups in the mid-twentieth century to nearly 90 percent representation from white, rural communities after 2010. There is heterogeneity across rural settings, however, with different parts of the country exhibiting region-specific trends in predominant drug types and rates of overdose.[6]

Given the persistent variability in potency and quality of illicit drugs and the ever-rising drug tolerance among people who use heroin, a third wave of overdose deaths commenced as dealers began to adulterate the heroin supply with fentanyl and fentanyl analogs to increase potency and profitability. In 2016 heroin deaths began to dip in the face of a new threat from fentanyl and its analogs nationwide. Fentanyl is a synthetic opioid at least fifty times more potent than heroin, and it is used by dealers at all levels as an adulterant to maintain or increase the potency of their merchandise after it has been cut, or diluted, with nonpsychoactive substances. Between 2013 and 2017 the presence of synthetic opioids other than methadone (predominantly fentanyl) in prescription opioid–related overdose deaths more than quadrupled, from 7.2 percent to more than 32 percent. During the same period, as heroin deaths were increasing in the United States, synthetic opioid involvement in mortality increased 1,980 percent, from 2.5 to 52.3 percent. Appalachian communities experienced an 817 percent rise in fentanyl-related mortality, a rate that was 72 percent higher than in the rest of the country between 2013 and 2017. In 2020 fentanyl caused more deaths than either heroin or prescription opioids.[7]

Surveillance of overdose mortality and its epidemiology is essential to understanding and predicting future trends in communities. Although surveillance is improving in some parts of Appalachia, it is difficult to ascertain how many nonfatal overdoses occur outside of those recorded by emergency medical services. In addition, it is impossible to determine the characteristics of the illicit drug market in real time so that overdose prevention efforts can be targeted where they are most needed. In the last three decades, the prevalence of OPR mortality has shifted dramatically upward and then flattened, with significant variations across the country. These changes often occur before the treatment community is aware of them and certainly before effective responses can be put in place.

Recognition of the Crisis as a Syndemic

Opioid addiction is associated with a multitude of social problems, such as increased crime, unemployment, legal issues, and trouble with interpersonal relationships. Rural Appalachia faces significant health disparities, and over the past fifty years, it has encountered diminishing economic opportunities and widening economic gaps; currently, its health statistics are worse than those in most of the rest of the country. As such, the opioid crisis is increasingly framed as a synergistic epidemic, or "syndemic," defined by Singer and colleagues in 2017 as "the aggregation of two or more diseases or other health conditions in a population in which there is some level of deleterious biological or behavior interface that exacerbates the negative health effects of any or all of the diseases involved." Syndemics result from multiple interrelated systems and processes that contribute to heightened vulnerability for disease.

Syndemic theory posits that some epidemics are sustained because of harmful social conditions and injurious social connections. For instance, increases in addiction, overdose, fatty liver disease, hepatitis C, HIV, neonatal abstinence syndrome, and suicide can be understood as syndemics driven by socioeconomic, corporate, cultural, and geographic forces.[8] Peters and colleagues, in elaborating on the "Hydra" of the opioid epidemic, conclude that:

> About 25 percent of counties nationally is severely impacted by opioid overdose fatalities, but not in the same manner as we identify distinct epidemics. The prescription opioid epidemic is the most common (8.9 percent of counties) and is overwhelmingly located in rural counties. A number of counties have transitioned to a synthetic-prescription mixture epidemic (6.9 percent), affecting both large urban cities and small rural places. The heroin epidemic is concentrated in the nation's larger metropolitan and smaller micropolitan cities (5.3 percent), but these illicit drugs are still relatively rare in rural counties. Lastly, a small share of counties (4.2 percent) are experiencing three coinciding epidemics of prescriptions, heroin, and synthetics—what we term an opioid overdose syndemic. Many central Appalachia counties suffer from an opioid syndemic, where the crisis began in the 1990s and has only worsened since.[9]

Simultaneously, opioid injection drug use is highly prevalent in Central Appalachia, where it is contributing to significant increases in hepatitis C and HIV infection. More than half (56 percent) of the counties deemed by the CDC to be most vulnerable to an outbreak of HIV lie within Central Appalachia. Rural counties in Appalachia exhibit high rates of overdose mortality, OPR sales, poor mental health, and other factors that make individuals highly vulnerable to both SUD and related infectious diseases. In addition, many Appalachian communities face high poverty and unemployment, geographic and social isolation, and the stigma associated with SUD, mental health problems, and HIV infection. These factors together contribute to limited access to services, low health literacy, and poor utilization of available services.[10]

Mitigation of the Opioid Crisis

Promising and evidence-based strategies exist to mitigate the devastating impacts of the opioid crisis. Strategies that can prevent and treat OUD, as well as reduce the harmful effects associated with OUD, are essential. Though not an exhaustive review, the following sections highlight a number of strategies, some of which may be crosscutting. Notably, a 2019 Appalachian Regional Commission (ARC) issue brief on opioid misuse in Appalachia provided multiple recommendations and practical strategies, some of which are elaborated on here. The opioid crisis cannot be solved rapidly or by a single strategy or sector. Persistent and coordinated implementation of promising and evidence-based strategies, with consideration of intended and unintended consequences, will help the region make measurable progress and advance public health.[11]

Prevention

Prevention strategies to mitigate the initiation of opioid misuse and progression to OUD can address the present opioid crisis and help avert future crises. Since the first wave of the opioid crisis, multiple strategies have been aimed at decreasing the supply of prescription opioids, and prescribing practices have been an important focus. According to Volkow and colleagues, "new federal guidelines and improved physician education in opioid prescribing and pain management are already having an influence on reducing overprescribing." For example, release of the CDC's guidelines for prescribing opioids for chronic pain in 2016 was associated with a change in various opioid prescribing practices (e.g., fewer high-dosage prescriptions). Similarly, PDMPs are a promising strategy. Implemented at the state level, PDMPs are electronic databases that collect data on dispensed controlled substances. Their characteristics differ across states, and although results have been mixed, PDMPs could improve opioid prescribing practices and reduce prescription opioid misuse and diversion, among other impacts. However, given the lethality of the two latest waves of the opioid crisis, interdiction strategies that can "interrupt the supply of heroin and illicitly produced synthetic opioids" are urgently needed.[12]

Alongside strategies aimed at decreasing the supply of opioids—both prescription and illicit—the demand for opioids must be reduced. Prevention interventions may be one such strategy that has the potential to mitigate all types of opioid misuse; however, research to strengthen the evidence specific to the *prevention* of opioid misuse is needed.[13] Evidence-based prevention interventions can be especially impactful among children and adolescents. Adolescence is a risky time of life for substance use initiation, and early substance use heightens the risk for the later development of SUDs. Effective programs that target underlying risk and protective factors can be implemented in family, school, or community settings. Evidence-based prevention interventions for young people, however, remain underused in the context of the opioid crisis.[14] Compton and colleagues concluded: "Reducing the risks of initiating opioid misuse by addressing modifiable childhood and adolescent risk and protective factors may be another 'ounce of prevention' that makes a substantial difference in a society and health care system now reeling from one of the worst drug crises our country has seen."[15]

Olsen and Sharfstein's *The Opioid Epidemic: What Everyone Needs to Know* provides an overview of the epidemic for a lay audience. They aptly describe the need for a "wide lens" approach to preventing addiction because the most effective programs call for skill development among youths prior to their exposure to drugs. Programs that have proved effective over many years include youth and community development approaches such as PROSPER and Communities that Care, which target youth skill acquisition to protect against multiple health threats. Additionally, numerous resources are available to support communities looking to implement evidence-based prevention approaches; these can be tailored to each community's specific setting and needs. One of the best places to find such programs is the Substance Abuse and Mental Health Services Administration's Evidence-Based Practices Resource Center.[16]

Treatment and Recovery

Because people with OUD have high rates of relapse, the most effective treatment involves maintenance on one of the three medications approved by the US Food and Drug Administration: methadone, buprenorphine, or naltrexone. Methadone and buprenorphine bind to opioid receptors in the brain (preventing withdrawal but not producing euphoria), while naltrexone blocks opioid receptors and prevents them from being activated. Collectively, these drugs are referred to as medications for opioid use disorder (MOUDs). They are effective in reducing illicit opioid use, opioid withdrawal symptoms, cravings, infectious disease transmission associated with needle use, risk for overdose, and criminal activity, as well as in increasing treatment compliance. Methadone must be provided by a licensed opioid treatment program or methadone clinic, while buprenorphine and naltrexone can be provided by physicians and other health care professionals (in the case of buprenorphine, a Drug Abuse Treatment Act of 2000 waiver is required). MOUDs are often administered in daily oral doses, although some are available as long-acting subdermal implants and injections, which reduce the patient's burden of daily dosing. In addition to medications, effective treatment programs for SUDs in general, including OUD, may include individual and/or group therapy, with a focus on building strong therapeutic alliances with patients. Programs for OUD may also be strengthened by the use of incentive-based approaches, such as offering small rewards for abstinence and treatment compliance, and by the treatment of common co-occurring conditions that impact compliance, including chronic pain, mood disorders, and infectious diseases.[17]

Despite considerable emphasis on the accessibility of MOUDs, the expansion of evidence-based treatment for OUD is required. One setting in dire need of OUD treatment is the criminal justice system. There are high rates of fatal opioid overdose among individuals transitioning from correctional facilities back into the community. Despite evidence that MOUDs provided during incarceration are effective in reducing illicit opioid use and increasing postrelease treatment, very few US jails and prisons offer this type of treatment. Offering MOUDs within the criminal justice system is one way to reach a sizable population of individuals with OUD who have a high risk of overdose and may not have access to treatment in their communities. There are several points in the justice system at which MOUDs could be administered, including upon diversion from incarceration (e.g., through drug treatment courts), throughout incarceration, and during community supervision after release. Similarly, reducing the stigma associated with OUD is another way to increase access to treatment. The characterization of OUD as a moral failing or a choice rather than a chronic disease, along with the belief that MOUDs allow individuals to "get high," discourages systems from offering MOUDs in the first place and can negatively influence provider-patient interactions. People stigmatized by OUD may be less likely to seek treatment. Ultimately, reducing barriers to the provision and receipt of MOUDs across various settings can facilitate the evidence-based treatment of OUD.[18]

It is important to know that recovery is possible. Recovery support services —"nonclinical services that assist individuals and families to recover from alcohol or drug problems"—can be beneficial and can be provided in various settings before, during, and after treatment. Evidence suggests that peer recovery support services can yield positive results, such as lower relapse rates. Similarly, the ARC's Substance Abuse Advisory Council proposed recovery ecosystems as a "sustainable solution" to the epidemic of substance misuse in Appalachia. A recovery ecosystem is a linkage of sectors (e.g., health care system, recovery communities, criminal justice system, employers) that helps individuals access the support services and training they need to maintain their recovery and attain employment. Given their posited role in increasing participation in the workforce and enhancing the region's economy, recovery ecosystems may be promising means of addressing structural factors that underlie the opioid crisis.[19]

Harm Reduction

Harm reduction strategies can also mitigate adverse outcomes associated with OUD, such as fatal overdose and infectious disease. For instance, naloxone is an opioid antagonist that can reverse the potentially deadly effects of opioid overdose and save lives. Improving access to naloxone has been an important focus of harm reduction strategies. The Office of the Surgeon General released a public health advisory on naloxone and opioid overdose in 2018 "to broaden the public awareness, availability, and use of life-saving naloxone to reduce opioid overdose mortality." Targeted distribution of naloxone to those at high risk for experiencing or observing an opioid overdose is one of the evidence-based strategies for preventing opioid overdose deaths. Methods to facilitate targeted distribution include instituting community-based programs, coprescribing naloxone and opioids, and supplying first responders with naloxone. Naloxone distribution can also be effective after a nonfatal overdose and offers an opportunity to connect overdose survivors with services. However, more research is needed to show how effective this is at preventing the long-term complications of OUD.[20]

Conversely, years of research support the effectiveness of comprehensive syringe services programs (SSPs). These community-based prevention programs can engage people who inject drugs and deliver a variety of valuable services, such as provision and disposal of syringes, provision of overdose prevention training and naloxone, and referral to treatment for SUDs, including MOUDs. SSPs can decrease the transmission of HIV and hepatitis C and contribute to other positive outcomes, such as fewer opioid overdose deaths. Taken together, a continued focus on improving access to effective harm reduction strategies is important for reducing OUD-related morbidity and mortality.[21]

In addition to providing services, SSPs can fill existing gaps in surveillance of OUD-related morbidity and mortality. They provide a touch point with a "hidden" community of people who inject drugs and may not otherwise be a part of routine surveillance activities. SSPs can monitor infectious disease prevalence as well as changes in the illicit drug market. Important work on how to analyze information from this type of hidden network is being conducted in Appalachian Kentucky. Similarly, an SSP in West Virginia leveraged its relationship with people who inject drugs to better understand the population. It found that the overwhelming majority were white, and nearly half were single males between the ages of thirty and thirty-nine. It was also able to determine clients' injection behaviors and their history of attempting to quit using drugs. In addition, it generated an estimate of the number of people who inject drugs, which can help legislators and public health officials allocate funds to support this hidden community. Enhanced surveillance could likewise facilitate targeted implementation and evaluation of evidence-based strategies.[22]

Summary and Recommendations

The opioid crisis that began in the late 1990s persists and has taken several forms over the decades. It is evolving even as these words are being read.

Methamphetamine use, alone and in combination with opioids, is surging in Appalachia and nationwide. Ellis and colleagues published a report demonstrating an 82 percent increase in past-month methamphetamine use among those attending outpatient methadone treatment programs in the six years from 2011 to 2017. Moreover, overdose deaths are increasingly attributed to both illicit opioids and psychostimulants, with one study showing a 42 percent increase in stimulant-related deaths from 2015 to 2016. This chapter has focused on opioids, but public health and other interested professionals are urged to think critically about the type and scale of community-level response required by an epidemic of this nature to achieve true and lasting mitigation. As history has shown, Appalachia is highly vulnerable to SUDs and associated complications. And although the opioid crisis has become national news, this was not always the case. Early reports about the crisis were interesting mainly to scholars and clinicians in the Appalachian region. It was many years before national-level agencies began to prioritize the crisis, and only then did funds start to flow to states for the implementation of evidence-based strategies.[23]

It is imperative for public health professionals, politicians, and others to be both vigilant and innovative in the coming years to mitigate the harms of the current crisis and prevent additional increases in overdose mortality in Appalachia and beyond. It is encouraging that community-level coalitions are rising up to address the epidemic, working with universities, industry, governmental stakeholders, and hospital systems in an increasingly coordinated fashion to implement best practices in the region. And it is encouraging that the National Institutes of Health's Helping to End Addiction Long-term (HEAL) initiative awarded three large, multiyear cooperative agreements to universities to focus on the systematic implementation of evidence-based approaches to the crisis in Appalachian communities. The list is too long to elaborate here, but innovations in sampling, epidemiology, rural access to care, hepatitis C and HIV risk mitigation, cost-effectiveness of scalable mental health treatment, sustainable platforms for prevention funding, university-community engagement, and university networks to maximize the impact of their research teams are all addressing the crisis in the region. The results are being disseminated widely, so the rest of the country and the world can learn from the Appalachian experience.

A colleague of ours was at the forefront of the HIV/AIDS crisis of the 1980s and 1990s. He has called HIV/AIDS the defining epidemic of his career, and the opioid crisis is the defining epidemic of the generation that followed him. The two crises share similarities, in that they proliferated largely among hidden groups that engaged in associated risky behaviors shrouded in stigma. Neither epidemic was challenged in a forthright and timely manner, which exacerbated their impacts. They are distinct in one very obvious way: the opioid crisis had corporate drivers and an apparatus of propagation that, on its face, was one of the most respected industries in the nation—the pharmaceutical companies and clinical medicine, respectively. We make no judgments about the intent of either the pharmaceutical industry or the medical profession relative to the crisis, but it is clear that both need greater oversight. The latter is being addressed iteratively with guidelines and training. The former is being adjudicated in courts across the nation, as opioid manufacturers, distributers, and dispensers are being sued by more than 2,000 cities, towns, states, health care systems, and individuals for their role in the crisis.[24]

Corporate drivers, hidden networks, and a health system and a public that have stigmatized both the condition and its treatment clearly point to the syndemic nature of the OUD crisis in Appalachia. But even the syndemic framing of OUD, as comprehensive as it is, does not capture the true costs to the Appalachian community. Regrettably, the region has felt the despair of families and friends and the cultural and economic impacts so acutely that the lessons learned in Appalachia have been collected, amplified, and told worldwide in every form of media. There is much to be learned here, and the great hope is that these lessons will be heeded by others before they feel the same impact.

Notes

1. Center for Behavioral Health Statistics and Quality, *2017 National Survey on Drug Use and Health: Detailed Tables* (Rockville, MD: SAMHSA, 2018), https://www.samhsa.gov/data/report/2017-nsduh-detailed-tables; Lawrence Scholl et al., "Drug and Opioid-Involved Overdose Deaths—United States, 2013–2017," *Morbidity and Mortality Weekly Report* 67, no. 5152 (2018): 1419–27; CDC, "Opioid Overdose: Understanding the Epidemic," reviewed March 19, 2020, https://www.cdc.gov/drugoverdose/epidemic/index.html; National Center for Health Statistics, "National Vital Statistics System," reviewed October 9, 2020, https://www.cdc.gov/nchs/nvss/index.htm; CDC, "CDC Wonder," reviewed November 5, 2020, https://wonder.cdc.gov; Karin A. Mack, Christopher M. Jones, and Michael F. Ballesteros, "Illicit Drug Use, Illicit Drug Use Disorders, and Drug Overdose Deaths in Metropolitan and Nonmetropolitan Areas—United States," *American Journal of Transplantation* 17, no. 12 (2017): 3241–52; Macarena C. Garcia et al., "Opioid Prescribing Rates in Nonmetropolitan and Metropolitan Counties among Primary Care Providers Using an Electronic Health Record System—United States, 2014–2017," *Morbidity and Mortality Weekly Report* 68, no. 2 (2019): 25–30; David J. Peters, Shannon M. Monnat, Andrew L. Hochstetler, and Mark T. Berg, "The Opioid Hydra: Understanding Overdose Mortality Epidemics and Syndemics across the Rural-Urban Continuum," *Rural Sociology* 85, no. 3 (2019): 589–622.

2. Pamela T. M. Leung, Erin M. Macdonald, Irfan A. Dhalla, and David N. Juurlink, "A 1980 Letter on the Risk of Opioid Addiction," *New England Journal of Medicine* 376, no. 22 (2017): 2194–95; Barry Meier, *A World of Hurt: Fixing Pain Medicine's Greatest Mistake*

(New York: New York Times Company, 2013); Russell K. Portenoy and Kathleen M. Foley, "Chronic Use of Opioid Analgesics in Non-malignant Pain: Report of 38 Cases," *Pain* 25, no. 2 (1986): 171–86.

3. CDC, "Vital Signs: Overdoses of Prescription Opioid Pain Relievers—United States, 1999–2008," *Morbidity and Mortality Weekly Report* 60, no. 43 (2011): 1487–92; Andrew Kolodny et al., "The Prescription Opioid and Heroin Crisis: A Public Health Approach to an Epidemic of Addiction," *Annual Review of Public Health* 36 (2015): 559–74; Lainie Rutkow, Jon S. Vernick, and G. Caleb Alexander, "More States Should Regulate Pain Management Clinics to Promote Public Health," *American Journal of Public Health* 107, no. 2 (2017): 240–43; S. C. Brighthaupt, E. M. Stone, L. Rutkow, and E. E. McGinty, "Effect of Pill Mill Laws on Opioid Overdose Deaths in Ohio & Tennessee: A Mixed-Methods Case Study," *Preventive Medicine* 126 (2019): 105736; Richard C. Dart et al., "Trends in Opioid Analgesic Abuse and Mortality in the United States," *New England Journal of Medicine* 372, no. 16 (2015): 1573–74; Scott Higham, Sari Horowitz, and Steven Rich, "76 Billion Opioid Pills: Newly Released Federal Data Unmasks the Epidemic," *Washington Post*, July 16, 2019, https://www.washingtonpost.com/investigations/76-billion-opioid-pills -newly-released-federal-data-unmasks-the-epidemic/2019/07/16/5f29fd62-a73e-11e9 -86dd-d7f0e60391e9_story.html.

4. Higham et al., "76 Billion Opioid Pills"; Zhiwei Zhang et al., *An Analysis of Mental Health and Substance Abuse Disparities and Access to Treatment Services in the Appalachian Region* (Washington, DC: NORC and ARC, 2008); Laura Moody, Emily Satterwhite, and Warren K. Bickel, "Substance Use in Rural Central Appalachia: Current Status and Treatment Considerations," *Rural Mental Health* 41, no. 2 (2017): 123–35; Leonard J. Paulozzi and Yongli Xi, "Recent Changes in Drug Poisoning Mortality in the United States by Urban-Rural Status and by Drug Type," *Pharmacoepidemiology and Drug Safety* 17, no. 10 (2008): 997–1005; Aron J. Hall et al., "Patterns of Abuse among Unintentional Pharmaceutical Overdose Fatalities," *JAMA* 300, no. 22 (2008): 2613–20.

5. Katherine M. Keyes et al., "Understanding the Rural-Urban Differences in Nonmedical Prescription Opioid Use and Abuse in the United States," *American Journal of Public Health* 104, no. 2 (2014): e52–59; Martha J. Wunsch et al., "Methadone-Related Overdose Deaths in Rural Virginia: 1997 to 2003," *Journal of Addiction Medicine* 7, no. 4 (2013): 223–29; Khary K. Rigg, Samantha J. March, and James A. Inciardi, "Prescription Drug Abuse & Diversion: Role of the Pain Clinic," *Journal of Drug Issues* 40, no. 3 (2010): 681–702; John J. Beggs, Valerie A. Haines, and Jeanna S. Hurlbert, "Revisiting the Rural-Urban Contrast: Personal Networks in Nonmetropolitan and Metropolitan Settings," *Rural Sociology* 61, no. 2 (1996): 306–25; Rand D. Conger and Glen H. Elder Jr., *Families in Troubled Times: Adapting to Change in Rural America; Social Institutions and Social Change* (New York: Aldine de Gruyter, 1994); Elizabeth Gorevski et al., "Utilization, Spending, and Price Trends for Benzodiazepines in the US Medicaid Program: 1991–2009," *Annals of Pharmacotherapy* 46, no. 4 (2012): 503–12; Mark D. Partridge and Dan S. Rickman, "High-Poverty Nonmetropolitan Counties in America: Can Economic Development Help?" *International Regional Science Review* 28, no. 4 (2005): 415–40.

6. Margaret Warner, Li Hui Chen, and Diane M. Makuc, "Increase in Fatal Poisonings Involving Opioid Analgesics in the United States, 1999–2006," *NCHS Data Brief* 22 (2009): 1–8; National Institute on Drug Abuse, "Overdose Death Rates," March 10, 2020, https:// www.drugabuse.gov/related-topics/trends-statistics/overdose-death-rates; CDC, "Opioid Overdose"; Kolodny et al., "Prescription Opioid and Herion Crisis"; Rigg et al., "Prescrip-

tion Drug Abuse"; Pradip K. Muhuri, Joseph C. Gfroerer, and M. Christine Davies, "Associations of Nonmedical Pain Reliever Use and Initiation of Heroin Use in the United States," *CBHSQ Data Review* (August 2013), https://www.samhsa.gov/data/sites/default/files /DR006/DR006/nonmedical-pain-reliever-use-2013.pdf; Theodore J. Cicreo et al., "The Changing Face of Heroin Use in the United States: A Retrospective Analysis of the Past 50 Years," *JAMA Psychiatry* 71, no. 7 (2014): 821–26.

7. Scholl et al., "Drug and Opioid-Involved Overdose Deaths"; CDC, "Opioid Overdose"; National Institute on Drug Abuse, "Overdose Death Rates"; Bryce Pardo et al., *The Future of Fentanyl and Other Synthetic Opioids* (Santa Monica, CA: RAND Corporation, 2019); National Association of Counties, "Opioids in Appalachia: The Role of Counties in Reversing a Regional Epidemic," 2019, https://www.naco.org/resources/featured/opioids -appalachia; DEA Strategic Intelligence Section, *2018 National Drug Threat Assessment* (Washington, DC: DEA and US Department of Justice, 2018); Julie K. O'Donnell et al., "Deaths Involving Fentanyl, Fentanyl Analogs, and U-47700—10 States, July–December 2016," *Morbidity and Mortality Weekly Report* 66, no. 43 (2017): 1197–202.

8. Jennifer C. Veilleux et al., "A Review of Opioid Dependence Treatment: Pharmacological and Psychosocial Interventions to Treat Opioid Addiction," *Clinical Psychology Review* 30, no. 2 (2010): 155–66; Adam Hege et al., "Social Determinants of Health and the Effects on Quality of Life and Well-being in 2 Rural Appalachia Communities: The Community Members" Perspective and Implications for Health Disparities," *Family & Community Health* 41, no. 4 (2018): 244–54; Elizabeth L. McGarvey et al., "Health Disparities between Appalachian and Non-Appalachian Counties in Virginia USA," *Journal of Community Health* 36, no. 3 (2011): 348–56; Gopal K. Singh, Michael D. Kogan, and Rebecca T. Slifkin, "Widening Disparities in Infant Mortality and Life Expectancy between Appalachia and the Rest of the United States, 1990-2013," *Health Affairs (Project Hope)* 36, no. 8 (2017): 1423; Brian N. Griffith, Gretchen D. Lovett, Donald N. Pyle, and Wayne C. Miller, "Self-Rated Health in Rural Appalachia: Health Perceptions Are Incongruent with Health Status and Health Behaviors," *BMC Public Health* 11, no. 229 (2011): 1–8; Michael Meit, Megan Heffernan, Erin Tanenbaum, and Topher Hoffman, *Final Report: Appalachian Diseases of Despair* (Washington, DC: NORC and ARC, 2017); Michael Morrone, Natalie A. Kruse, and Amy E. Chadwick, "Environmental and Health Disparities in Appalachian Ohio: Perceptions and Realities," *Journal of Health Disparities Research and Practice* 7, no. 5 (2014): 5; Merrill Singer, Nicola Bulled, Bayla Ostrach, and Emily Mendenhall, "Syndemics and the Biosocial Conception of Health," *Lancet* 389, no. 10072 (2017): 941–50; Patrick A. Wilson et al., "Using Syndemic Theory to Understand Vulnerability to HIV Infection among Black and Latino Men in New York City," *Journal of Urban Health* 91, no. 5 (2014): 983–98; Merrill Singer and Scott Clair, "Syndemics and Public Health: Reconceptualizing Disease in Biosocial Context," *Medical Anthropology Quarterly* 17, no. 4 (2003): 423–41.

9. Peters et al., "Opioid Hydra."

10. Jon E. Zibbell et al., "Increases in Hepatitis C Virus Infection Related to Injection Drug Use among Persons Aged ≤30 Years—Kentucky, Tennessee, Virginia, and West Virginia, 2006–2012," *Morbidity and Mortality Weekly Report* 64, no. 17 (2015): 453–58; Michelle M. Van Handel et al., "County-Level Vulnerability Assessment for Rapid Dissemination of HIV or HCV Infections among Persons Who Inject Drugs, United States," *Journal of Acquired Immune Deficiency Syndromes* 73, no. 3 (2016): 323–31; T. G. Heckman et al., "Barriers to Care among Persons Living with HIV/AIDS in Urban and Rural Areas," *AIDS Care* 10, no. 3 (1998): 365–75; S. Reif, C. E. Golin, and S. R. Smith, "Barriers to

Accessing HIV/AIDS Care in North Carolina: Rural and Urban Differences," *AIDS Care* 17, no. 5 (2005): 558–65.

11. Kolodny et al., "Prescription Opioid and Heroin Crisis"; G. Caleb Alexander, Shannon Frattaroli, and Andrea Gielen, eds., *The Opioid Epidemic: From Evidence to Impact* (Baltimore: Johns Hopkins Bloomberg School of Public Health, 2017); Nora D. Volkow et al., "Prevention and Treatment of Opioid Misuse and Addiction: A Review," *JAMA Psychiatry* 76, no. 2 (2019): 208–16; Wilson M. Compton, Maureen Boyle, and Eric Wargo, "Prescription Opioid Abuse: Problems and Responses," *Preventive Medicine* 80 (2015): 5–9; ETSU and NORC, *Issue Brief: Health Disparities Related to Opioid Misuse in Appalachia: Practical Strategies and Recommendations for Communities* (Washington, DC: ARC, 2019), https://www.arc.gov/wp-content/uploads/2020/06/HealthDisparitiesRelatedtoOpioidMisuseinAppalachiaApr2019.pdf; National Academies of Sciences, Engineering, and Medicine, "Evidence on Strategies for Addressing the Opioid Epidemic," in *Pain Management and the Opioid Epidemic: Balancing Societal and Individual Benefits and Risks of Prescription Opioid Use,* ed. M. A. Ford and R. J. Bonnie (Washington, DC: National Academies Press, 2017), 267–358; Wilson M. Compton et al., "Targeting Youth to Prevent Later Substance Use Disorder: An Underutilized Response to the US Opioid Crisis," *American Journal of Public Health* 109, no. S3 (2019): S185–89; Stephanie M. Mathis et al., "A Dissemination and Implementation Science Approach to the Epidemic of Opioid Use Disorder in the United States," *Current HIV/AIDS Reports* 15, no. 5 (2018): 359–70; Tamara M. Haegerich et al., "Evidence for State, Community and Systems-Level Prevention Strategies to Address the Opioid Crisis," *Drug and Alcohol Dependence* 204 (2019): 107563; Andrew Kolodny and Thomas R. Frieden, "Ten Steps the Federal Government Should Take Now to Reverse the Opioid Addiction Epidemic," *JAMA* 318, no. 16 (2017): 1537–38; Kathryn F. Hawk, Federico E. Vaca, and Gail D'Onofrio, "Reducing Fatal Opioid Overdose: Prevention, Treatment and Harm Reduction Strategies," *Yale Journal of Biology and Medicine* 88, no. 3 (2015): 235–45; Daniel Ciccarone, "The Triple Wave Epidemic: Supply and Demand Drivers of the US Opioid Overdose Crisis," *International Journal on Drug Policy* 71 (2019): 183–88.

12. Mathis et al., "Dissemination and Implementation"; Ciccarone, "Triple Wave Epidemic"; Volkow et al., "Prevention and Treatment"; Nora Volkow, "The Importance of Prevention in Addressing the Opioid Crisis," *Nora's Blog* by the National Institute on Drug Abuse, June 27, 2019, https://www.drugabuse.gov/about-nida/noras-blog/2019/06/importance-prevention-in-addressing-opioid-crisis; Compton et al., "Prescription Opioid Abuse"; Compton et al., "Targeting Youth"; Theodore J. Cicero, Zachary A. Kasper, and Matthew S. Ellis, "Increased Use of Heroin as an Initiating Opioid of Abuse," *Addictive Behaviors* 74 (2017): 63–66; Rosalie Liccardo Pacula and David Powell, "A Supply-Side Perspective on the Opioid Crisis," *Journal of Policy Analysis and Management* 37, no. 2 (2018): 438–46; Deborah Dowell, Tamara M. Haegerich, and Roger Chou, "CDC Guideline for Prescribing Opioids for Chronic Pain—United States, 2016," *Morbidity and Mortality Weekly Report* 65, no. 1 (2016): 1–49; Amy S. B. Bohnert, Gery P. Guy Jr., and Jan L. Losby, "Opioid Prescribing in the United States before and after the Centers for Disease Control and Prevention's 2016 Opioid Guideline," *Annals of Internal Medicine* 169, no. 6 (2018): 367–75; CDC, "What States Need to Know about PDMPs," reviewed June 10, 2020, https://www.cdc.gov/drugoverdose/pdmp/states.html; Tamara M. Haegerich, Leonard J. Paulozzi, Brian J. Manns, and Christopher M. Jones, "What We Know, and Don't Know, about the Impact of State Policy and Systems-Level Interventions on Prescription Drug Overdose," *Drug and Alcohol Dependence* 145 (2014): 34–47; Janet Weiner, Yuhua Bao, and Zachary Meisel, *Issue Brief: Prescription Drug Monitoring Programs; Evolution*

and Evidence (Philadelphia: Penn Leonard Davis Institute of Health Economics, 2017), https://ldi.upenn.edu/brief/prescription-drug-monitoring-programs-evolution-and-evidence; *Briefing on PDMP Effectiveness* (PDMP Center of Excellence at Brandeis University, 2014), http://www.akleg.gov/basis/get_documents.asp?session=29&docid=63914; Erin P. Finley et al., "Evaluating the Impact of Prescription Drug Monitoring Program Implementation: A Scoping Review," *BMC Health Services Research* 17, no. 1 (2017): 420; National Institute on Drug Abuse, "Policy Brief: Improving Opioid Prescribing," March 2017, https://www.drugabuse.gov/publications/improving-opioid-prescribing/improving-opioid-prescribing; SAMHSA, "Prescription Drug Monitoring Programs: A Guide for Healthcare Providers," *In Brief* 10, no. 1 (2017), https://store.samhsa.gov/product/In-Brief-Prescription-Drug-Monitoring-Programs-A-Guide-for-Healthcare-Providers/SMA16-4997; Kolodny and Frieden, "Ten Steps."

13. Volkow et al., "Prevention and Treatment"; Compton et al., "Prescription Opioid Abuse"; Compton et al., "Targeting Youth"; Volkow, "Importance of Prevention."

14. Compton et al., "Targeting Youth"; Chloe J. Jordan and Susan L. Andersen, "Sensitive Periods of Substance Abuse: Early Risk for the Transition to Dependence," *Developmental Cognitive Neuroscience* 25 (2017): 29–44; Kenneth W. Griffin and Gilbert J. Botvin, "Evidence-Based Interventions for Preventing Substance Use Disorders in Adolescents," *Child and Adolescent Psychiatric Clinics of North America* 19, no. 3 (2010): 505–26; Dawn L. Thatcher and Duncan B. Clark, "Adolescents at Risk for Substance Use Disorders: Role of Psychological Dysregulation, Endophenotypes, and Environmental Influences," *Alcohol Research & Health* 31, no. 2 (2008): 168–76; Volkow et al., "Prevention and Treatment"; Mathis et al., "Dissemination and Implementation"; US Department of Health and Human Services (DHHS), Office of the Surgeon General, *Facing Addiction in America: The Surgeon General's Spotlight on Opioids* (Washington, DC: DHHS, 2018), https://addiction.surgeongeneral.gov/sites/default/files/Spotlight-on-Opioids_09192018.pdf; Elizabeth B. Robertson, Susan L. David, and Suman A. Rao, *Preventing Drug Use among Children and Adolescents: A Research-Based Guide for Parents, Educators, and Community Leaders*, NIH Publication no. 04-4212(A) (Bethesda, MD: National Institute on Drug Abuse, National Institutes of Health, and US Department of Health and Human Services, 2003).

15. Compton et al., "Targeting Youth."

16. Yngvild Olsen and Joshua M. Sharfstein, *The Opioid Epidemic: What Everyone Needs to Know* (New York: Oxford University Press, 2019); Partnerships in Prevention Science Institute, "PROSPER Partnerships," http://helpingkidsprosper.org/; University of Washington Center for Communities that Care, "Communities that Care PLUS," https://www.communitiesthatcare.net/; SAMHSA, Evidence-Based Practices Resource Center, updated April 30, 2020, https://www.samhsa.gov/ebp-resource-center.

17. Volkow et al., "Prevention and Treatment"; Alan I. Leshner and Michelle Mancher, eds., *Medications for Opioid Use Disorder Save Lives* (Washington, DC: National Academies Press, 2019); Catherine Anne Fullerton et al., "Medication-Assisted Treatment with Methadone: Assessing the Evidence," *Psychiatric Services* 65, no. 2 (2014): 146–57; Richard P. Mattick, Courtney Breen, Jo Kimber, and Marina Davoli, "Methadone Maintenance Therapy versus No Opioid Replacement Therapy for Opioid Dependence," *Cochrane Database of Systematic Reviews* 3, no. 2 (2009); Walter Ling et al., "Buprenorphine Implants for Treatment of Opioid Dependence: A Randomized Controlled Trial," *JAMA* 304, no. 14 (2010): 1576–83; Lars Tanum et al., "Effectiveness of Injectable Extended-Release Naltrexone vs Daily Buprenorphine-Naloxone for Opioid Dependence: A Randomized Clinical Noninferiority Trial," *JAMA Psychiatry* 74, no. 12 (2017): 1197–205; Christine Timko et al., "Retention in

Medication-Assisted Treatment for Opiate Dependence: A Systematic Review," *Journal of Addictive Diseases* 35, no. 1 (2016): 22–35; *Principles of Drug Addiction Treatment: A Research-Based Guide* (Washington, DC: National Institute on Drug Abuse, 2012), https://www.drugabuse.gov/sites/default/files/podat_1.pdf; National Institute on Drug Abuse, "Medications to Treat Opioid Use Disorder," updated June 2018, https://www.drugabuse.gov/publications/research-reports/medications-to-treat-opioid-use-disorder.

18. *Principles of Drug Abuse Treatment for Criminal Justice Populations: A Research-Based Guide* (Washington, DC: National Institute on Drug Abuse, 2014), https://www.drugabuse.gov/sites/default/files/txcriminaljustice_0.pdf; Ingrid A. Binswanger, Patrick J. Blatchford, Shane R. Mueller, and Marc F. Stern, "Mortality after Prison Release: Opioid Overdose and Other Causes of Death, Risk Factors, and Time Trends from 1999 to 2009," *Annals of Internal Medicine* 159, no. 9 (2013): 592–600; Elizabeth C. Merrall et al., "Meta-analysis of Drug-Related Deaths Soon after Release from Prison," *Addiction* 105, no. 9 (2010): 1545–54; Kelley E. Moore et al., "Effectiveness of Medication Assisted Treatment for Opioid Use in Prison and Jail Settings: A Meta-analysis and Systematic Review," *Journal of Substance Abuse Treatment* 99 (2019): 32–43; Anjalee Sharma et al., "Pharmacotherapy for Opioid Dependence in Jails and Prisons: Research Review Update and Future Directions," *Substance Abuse Rehabilitation* 7 (2016): 27–40; Sarah E. Wakeman and Josiah D. Rich, "Addiction Treatment within U.S. Correctional Facilities: Bridging the Gap between Current Practice and Evidence-Based Care," *Journal of Addictive Diseases* 34, no. 2–3 (2015): 220–25; SAMHSA, *Use of Medication-Assisted Treatment for Opioid Use Disorder in Criminal Justice Settings* (Rockville, MD: US Department of Health and Human Services, 2019), https://store.samhsa.gov/product/Use-of-Medication-Assisted-Treatment-for-Opioid-Use-Disorder-in-Criminal-Justice-Settings/PEP19-MATUSECJS; Yngvild Olsen and Joshua M. Sharfstein, "Confronting the Stigma of Opioid Use Disorder—and Its Treatment," *JAMA* 311, no. 14 (2014): 1393–94; Sarah E. Wakeman and Josiah D. Rich, "Barriers to Medications for Addiction Treatment: How Stigma Kills," *Substance Use & Misuse* 53, no. 2 (2018): 330–33; Lawrence H. Yang et al., "A New Brief Opioid Stigma Scale to Assess Perceived Public Attitudes and Internalized Stigma: Evidence for Construct Validity," *Journal of Substance Abuse Treatment* 99 (2019): 44–51; Julia Woo et al., "'Don't Judge a Book by Its Cover': A Qualitative Study of Methadone Patients' Experiences of Stigma," *Substance Abuse: Research and Treatment* 11 (2017): 1178221816685087.

19. DHHS, *Facing Addiction in America;* Linda Kaplan, *The Role of Recovery Support Services in Recovery-Oriented Systems of Care*, DHHS Publication no. (SMA) 08-4315 (Rockville, MD: Center for Substance Abuse Treatment, SAMHSA, 2008); ARC Substance Abuse Advisory Council, *Report of Recommendations: Appalachian Regional Commission's Substance Abuse Advisory Council* (Washington, DC: ARC, 2019), https://www.arc.gov/wp-content/uploads/2020/06/SAAC-ReportofRecommendations-Sept2019.pdf.

20. National Institute on Drug Abuse, "Naloxone for Opioid Overdose: Life-Saving Science," 2017, https://www.drugabuse.gov/publications/naloxone-opioid-overdose-life-saving-science/naloxone-opioid-overdose-life-saving-science; DHHS, "US Surgeon General's Advisory on Naloxone and Opioid Overdose," updated April 5, 2019, https://www.hhs.gov/surgeongeneral/priorities/opioids-and-addiction/naloxone-advisory/index.html; Jennifer J. Carroll, Traci C. Green, and Rita K. Noonan, *Evidence-Based Strategies for Preventing Opioid Overdose: What's Working in the United States* (Washington, DC: CDC, 2018), https://www.cdc.gov/drugoverdose/pdf/pubs/2018-evidence-based-strategies.pdf; Jerome M. Adams, "Increasing Naloxone Awareness and Use: The Role of Health Care Prac-

titioners," *JAMA* 319, no. 20 (2018): 2073–74; Sarah M. Bagley, Samantha F. Schoenberger, Katherine M. Waye, and Alexander Y. Walley, "A Scoping Review of Post Opioid-Overdose Interventions," *Preventive Medicine* 128 (2019): 105813.

21. CDC, "Summary of Information on the Safety and Effectiveness of Syringe Services Programs (SSPs)," reviewed May 23, 2019, https://www.cdc.gov/ssp/syringe-services -programs-summary.html; CDC, "Syringe Services Programs (SSPs) Fact Sheet," reviewed May 23, 2019, https://www.cdc.gov/ssp/syringe-services-programs-factsheet.html; Carroll et al., *Evidence-Based Strategies.*

22. Abby E. Rudolph, April M. Young, and Jennifer R. Havens, "Examining the Social Context of Injection Drug Use: Social Proximity to Persons Who Inject Drugs versus Geographic Proximity to Persons Who Inject Drugs," *American Journal of Epidemiology* 186, no. 8 (2017): 970–78; Abby E. Rudolph, April M. Young, and Jennifer R. Havens, "Using Network and Spatial Data to Better Target Overdose Prevention Strategies in Rural Appalachia," *Journal of Urban Health* 96, no. 1 (2019): 27–37; April M. Young, Abby E. Rudolph, and Jennifer R. Havens, "Network-Based Research on Rural Opioid Use: An Overview of Methods and Lessons Learned," *Current HIV/AIDS Reports* 15, no. 2 (2018): 113–19; April M. Young, Abby E. Rudolph, Deane Quillen, and Jennifer R. Havens, "Spatial, Temporal and Relational Patterns in Respondent-Driven Sampling: Evidence from a Social Network Study of Rural Drug Users," *Journal of Epidemiology and Community Health* 68, no. 8 (2014): 792–98; Sean T. Allen et al., "Estimating the Number of People Who Inject Drugs in a Rural County in Appalachia," *American Journal of Public Health* 109, no. 3 (2019): 445–50.

23. Matthew S. Ellis, Zachary A. Kasper, and Theodore J. Cicero, "Twin Epidemics: The Surging Rise of Methamphetamine Use in Chronic Opioid Users," *Drug and Alcohol Dependence* 193 (2018): 14–20; R. Matt Gladden, Julie O'Donnell, Christine L. Mattson, and Puja Seth, "Changes in Opioid-Involved Overdose Deaths by Opioid Type and Presence of Benzodiazepines, Cocaine, and Methamphetamine—25 States, July–December 2017 to January–June 2018," *Morbidity and Mortality Weekly Report* 68, no. 34 (2019): 737–44; Mbabazi Kariisa et al., "Drug Overdose Deaths Involving Cocaine and Psychostimulants with Abuse Potential—United States, 2003–2017," *Morbidity and Mortality Weekly Report* 68, no. 17 (2019): 388–95.

24. Abbe R. Gluck, Ashley Hall, and Gregory Curfman, "Civil Litigation and the Opioid Epidemic: The Role of Courts in a National Health Crisis," *Journal of Law, Medicine & Ethics* 46, no. 2 (2018): 351–66; Cheryl Healton, "The Tobacco Master Settlement Agreement— Strategic Lessons for Addressing Public Health Problems," *New England Journal of Medicine* 379, no. 11 (2018): 997–1000; James G. Hodge and Lawrence O. Gostin, "Guiding Industry Settlements of Opioid Litigation," *American Journal of Drug and Alcohol Abuse* 45, no. 5 (2019): 432–37; Jeffrey Mervis, "First Opioid Settlement Lets Researchers Think Big," *Science* 364, no. 6435 (2019): 11–12.

10

Public Health Preparedness in Appalachia

MARGARET A. RIGGS AND JAMES ALAN RILEY

People rarely think about how to protect and improve community health and well-being through prevention until a public health crisis captures their attention. In 2020 the importance of public health preparedness—the field of science that works to prevent or reduce the impacts of public health emergencies—was underscored by a small virus that shut down the world. History has demonstrated that humankind cannot avoid communicable diseases, despite scientific advances. As Ong and Heymann put it, this "timeless dance" between humans and microbes began long ago and will continue far into the future. Microbes constantly evolve as a survival mechanism, and these organisms have adapted to exploit opportunities to spread to humans from the environment, from animals, or from other humans, causing novel diseases such as Ebola, Zika, and now COVID-19. Whether caused by a microbe, a weather event, or man-made circumstances, disasters occur, and the steps that governments, societies, and local communities take to avoid them—or, more importantly, to reduce their impact—are key to community health and resiliency.[1]

Natural disasters, disease outbreaks, and other public health emergencies can have widespread and long-lasting effects on supplies and services. These events fall into the hazard cycle, which is characterized by four temporal states: preparedness, mitigation, response, and recovery. Lessons learned during past public health disasters—such as 9/11, Hurricane Katrina, and the 2009 H1N1 influenza pandemic—have led to changes in the ways disasters and hazards are managed. According to the Federal Emergency Management Agency (FEMA), every response is local, as are many of the resources required to manage the response. Since 9/11, the Public Health Emergency Preparedness (PHEP) program of the Centers for Disease Control and Prevention (CDC) has partnered with state, local, tribal, and territorial public health departments to prepare and plan for emergencies. Health departments must be able to handle many different types of emergencies that threaten the health and safety of families and communities. PHEP supports sixty-two public health departments across the nation (in all fifty states and eight US territories) to protect Americans and save lives. PHEP is important to local preparedness and response because it builds community resilience. Mitigation research also suggests that, to improve resilience, policies should require the adoption of hazard reduction measures, rather than allowing them to be voluntary. Although implementing these policies and steps is the responsibility of local leaders, they may not have the resources necessary to do so. Fiscal challenges are often most intense at the local level, especially in small, rural Appalachian communities.[2]

Public health emergencies such as infectious disease outbreaks and natural disasters require a coordinated response by a wide range of community partners. Disasters are often portrayed in the media as discrete, abnormal events, but this characterization fails to account for communities' role in preparing for emergencies and building resiliency. The overall message to the public is that since disasters are inevitable events, the best recourse is to cope with them, clean up, provide relief, recover, and move on. Public health officials throughout the United States learned a number of valuable lessons from the practical application of community messaging, and the efforts used to mitigate flooding in New Orleans following Hurricane Katrina in 2005 are applicable to the COVID-19 pandemic. When the emergency is over, public interest fades—until the cycle resumes with the next disaster. Therefore, before a disaster hits, creating multijurisdictional coalitions and plans, developing risk communication strategies, rehearsing a unified incident command, and involving the local community are essential for effective preparedness.[3]

A community's health and resilience influence its ability to prepare for and recover from disasters. To build resilience, healthy communities must focus on the prevention of chronic illness. However, the US health care system generally concentrates on the management of acute disease episodes rather than on prevention. Although low-tech methods of preventive care, exercise, and sound nutrition lead to healthier communities, treating illness often takes precedence over promoting health. A healthier community is a more resilient community when disaster strikes. Populations in Appalachia have high rates of underlying health conditions, which makes them more likely to experience adverse health outcomes during an emergency. The health disparities in Appalachia highlight the need for a greater focus on health and prevention before an emergency strikes (see chapter 3 for more details on health disparities in Appalachia). Building health and resilience *before* a disaster can mitigate adverse outcomes.[4]

Appalachia—a region known primarily for its great mountain ranges—encompasses many different landforms: forested mountains, sloping ridges that lead to hidden hollows, and meandering rivers that travel through small towns. As chapter 2 explains, Appalachian towns are filled with tight-knit groups of people who are heterogenous yet have strong cultural ties. The federally defined region of Appalachia is divided into five subregions with differing demographics and health challenges (see chapters 3 and 4): Northern, North Central, Central, South Central, and Southern. The region is known for traditional music and self-reliant, diverse, strong-willed communities that remain fiercely independent despite limited economic opportunities and pervasive poverty. The remoteness of the forested mountains and hollows provides a sense of insulation from the outside world. Most parts of Appalachia get few visitors and have low population densities, which may slow the impact of natural disasters. This region is rich in coal, iron, and natural gas and has acres of harvestable timber, but it is also subject to a wide variety of natural disasters, such as tornadoes, floods, and mud slides, as well as a number of man-made disasters (see chapter 7).[5]

Public emergencies—whether resulting from man-made or natural disasters—have long challenged Appalachian communities. In recent years, regional infrastructure has been tested by a number of emergencies: the 2008 Kingston TVA coal ash spill in Tennessee; the 2012 tornado outbreak in eastern Kentucky; and train derailments in 2014 and 2015 that resulted in fires or contamination of waterways in Lynchburg (Virginia), the Elk River (West Virginia), and Fayette County (West Virginia). As recently as February 2020, a rock slide approximately 300 feet long and 50 feet wide caused a ninety-six-car train derailment in Draffin, Kentucky; five of those cars were carrying ethanol, which spilled into the Big Sandy River and subsequently caught fire. Water intake valves were located only a few miles downstream, and the incident affected the water supply of several surrounding communities. Such events are localized and limited in scope, and they might not make the national news, but they can be devastating to Appalachian residents. Given the potentially long-lasting health consequences of such disasters, the use of emergency preparedness plans to prevent or minimize the impact of future threats is critical to public health.[6]

Of course, the most pressing concern at the time of this writing is the still-unfolding COVID-19 pandemic. In 2020 Appalachia was neither protected nor insulated from the effects of COVID-19, a newly emerging disease first identified in Wuhan, China, in December 2019 that led to a worldwide pandemic. Severe acute respiratory syndrome coronavirus 2 (SARS-CoV-2), the virus that causes COVID-19, had not previously been identified in humans. It causes respiratory illness and can be spread from person to person. Prevention of newly emerging diseases such as COVID-19 is particularly challenging in places with high levels of poverty, geographic isolation, and low resource availability. Central Appalachia—comprising southwestern West Virginia, eastern Kentucky, southwestern Virginia, eastern Tennessee, and western North Carolina—struggles with poverty, geographic isolation, and limited public resources. Not surprisingly, the COVID-19 pandemic tested (and is still testing)

Appalachia's resilience and public health preparedness in these areas. This chapter explores the public health response in the early stages of the outbreak to better understand the roles of public health surveillance and planning in building and strengthening healthy, resilient communities across the region.[7]

Appalachia's Pandemic Response

As COVID-19 spread across the globe and quickly made its way to the United States, rural Appalachian communities did not feel the initial impact as harshly as others did. Many small Central Appalachian counties did not see their first cases until mid-May 2020, nearly two months after the virus was impacting large, urban areas of the United States. However, when the first cases appeared in the United States, small, rural Appalachian public health departments, aware of the health disparities within their communities, kept a watchful eye and took action to prevent the spread of the virus.[8]

The pandemic may take a greater toll on rural areas if their unique socioeconomic, sociomedical, and sociopolitical needs are not considered. For 2021, the Appalachian Regional Commission (ARC), employing an index-based classification system using three-year averages of economic indicators (unemployment rate, per capita market income, and poverty rate), identified seventy-eight counties as "distressed"—that is counties with higher poverty or lower income levels than national averages that rank in the worst 10 percent of the nation—with more than 65 percent of those counties found in Central Appalachia. Forty-two percent of the Appalachian region's population is rural, compared with 20 percent of the US population. The largely remote Appalachian region's challenges related to accessing quality health care, combined with its numerous health disparities, put the population at high risk for poor outcomes.[9]

Some people who develop COVID-19 become seriously ill and experience complications that can lead to death; the risk of severe disease increases steadily with age. People in the Appalachian region are at risk of developing serious complications from COVID-19. The proportion of the population aged sixty-five years and older exceeded the national average by more than two percentage points in 2018 (18.4 versus 16 percent). Additionally, people of all ages with underlying medical conditions (e.g., cancer; chronic kidney disease; chronic obstructive pulmonary disease; obesity; immunocompromised state due to solid organ transplantation; serious heart conditions such as heart failure, coronary artery disease, and cardiomyopathies; sickle cell disease; and type 2 diabetes) appear to be at higher risk of developing severe COVID-19 illness than those without these conditions. An estimated 60 percent of American adults have at least one chronic medical condition, and this percentage is higher among adults in the Appalachian region (see chapters 3 and 4). Obesity (body mass index of 30 or higher) is one of the most common underlying conditions that can increase the risk of severe COVID-19 illness. As of 2018, more than 42 percent of US adults were obese, and more than 9 percent were severely obese. Appalachian counties consistently have a high incidence of obesity (discussed in more detail in chapter 3). The more underlying medical conditions a person has, the higher the risk of developing severe complications from COVID-19. As CDC data show, hospitalization rates rise as the number of underlying health conditions increases, and the likelihood of hospitalization and death increases with age.[10]

Tried-and-true public health measures—used before vaccines became widely available and after the emergence of variants—have helped slow the spread of COVID-19. These measures included contact tracing, social distancing, and even one of the basic prevention methods used during the 1918 influenza pandemic: face masks. Pike County, Kentucky (population 58,000+), located in the eastern corner of the state, announced its first COVID-19 case on March 31, 2020. Before then, the Pike County COVID-19 Task Force had been meeting almost daily at the Pike County Health Department to prepare for COVID-19, after learning of the proverbial "canary in a coal mine" situations in other hard-hit areas of the United States. The task force was diligent about keeping the public informed and promoting drive-through testing, social distancing, and mask wearing. In neighboring Mingo County (population 23,000+), located in south-central West Virginia, the first COVID-19 case was identified on April 15, 2020. By that date, eleven of the fifty-five counties in West Virginia still had zero cases of COVID-19. Before that first positive case was announced, the Mingo County Health Department took early action and collaborated with the local community hospital to arrange a drive-through testing site, for which the hospital provided test kits and other supplies.[11]

Challenges in Appalachia

Disasters pose greater threats to communities that lack resources and access to health care, which are precursors to health disparities. Rural Appalachia's declining public health infrastructure and lack of access to public health professionals have made response and recovery efforts more challenging. Many Appalachian counties have experienced a long-term shortage of health care professionals, and residents may need to travel great distances to get treatment at specialized health care referral centers. If left untreated, chronic health problems can quickly become acute, and they have been linked to increased mortality among vulnerable populations in the wake of a disaster. As Behringer and Friedell note, the

Appalachian region's number of physically unhealthy days, number of mentally unhealthy days, and prevalence of depression are all higher than the national averages (a fact confirmed by the analysis in chapter 3). The region also has fewer health care professionals, lower average household incomes, and higher rates of poverty, obesity, smoking, and physical inactivity than the nation overall.[12]

Gaining the public's trust to follow public health recommendations is also a challenge in the region. During the investigation of a recent rabies outbreak in West Virginia, communication between the health department and its partners was identified as a strength in rural areas, but communication with the public was identified as a potential barrier. Due to the area's low population density and rural nature, it was challenging to get up-to-date information to people and to conduct disease surveillance activities. Low socioeconomic status and limited telecommunications infrastructure in the region also posed barriers, as many people lacked easy access to the internet. Barring improvements to the telecommunications infrastructure, website updates as the only means of reaching and educating the public may be insufficient. More traditional means of communication, such as in-person meetings, radio, television, and newspapers, may be necessary, in addition to using social media.[13]

The importance of religion in Appalachian culture is well documented, and Appalachians consider both faith and the benefits of medical care when seeking solutions to health problems, as Crainshaw notes. Actions and beliefs in Appalachia are based largely on discussions among community members about their personal experiences with disease and health care. A better understanding of the balance of such influences in Appalachia is critical to improving public health messaging. Although Appalachian individuals are known for being fiercely independent, self-reliant, and slow to trust, during the COVID-19 pandemic, they often listened to their personal health care providers about the importance of social isolation and the need to change precious traditions such as funerals and in-person church services. Communication among patients, health professionals, and faith leaders is instrumental in creating trust, which is the critical factor in an individual's acceptance of information and the use of mitigation strategies. If public health professionals acknowledge these characteristics of the people of Appalachia, they might enable more effective two-way communication. Reaching people where they are by using the knowledge of local thought leaders is key to gaining trust.[14]

Making a Difference in Appalachia

Public health preparedness is intertwined with individual health and resilience. These factors are important because healthy, socially connected, prepared individuals make stronger, more resilient communities that are better able to withstand, manage, and recover from disasters. A community resilience approach expands traditional preparedness efforts by promoting strong community systems and addressing the many factors that contribute to health. Community resilience is the sustained ability to withstand, adapt to, and recover from adversity, and, as the Department of Health and Human Services notes, "health—meaning physical, behavioral, social, and environmental health and wellbeing—is a big part of overall resilience." A resilient community is socially connected and has accessible health systems that are able to withstand disaster and foster community recovery. A resilient community can take collective action after an adverse event because it has developed resources that reduce the impact of major disturbances and protect people's health. It promotes individual and community health—physical, behavioral, and social—to strengthen the community to meet daily challenges as well as emergencies.[15] Many efforts to build resilient communities are already under way in Appalachia, including the following:

- **The Health Wagon:** Strong day-to-day systems can be leveraged to support health resilience during disasters and emergencies. The Health Wagon (see chapter 5) recognized that its patients' underlying health conditions put them at increased risk for complications from COVID-19, so it rapidly expanded its ability to conduct SARS-CoV-2 testing and to make referrals for social services through local health departments.[16]
- **Active Southern West Virginia (SWV):** Information and education related to public health, behavioral health, emergency preparedness, and community health resilience interventions can help people face everyday challenges as well as major disruptions or disasters. Optimal levels of physical and psychological health and well-being within the population can facilitate the community's rapid recovery from adverse events. In response to CDC guidance aimed at curbing the spread of COVID-19, after-school activities, including the Active SWV Kids Run Clubs, were canceled. To ensure that children retained some of the structure and support provided by playing sports, Active SWV launched a virtual edition of its spring 2020 Kids Run Club program. The students participated in Kids Run Club activities from home and logged their time with a free online tracking app that also allowed them to see what others from their school were doing. Active SWV urged participants to do their part to prevent the spread of COVID-19 by maintaining safe distances; washing hands often with soap and water for at least twenty seconds; avoiding touching their

eyes, nose, and mouth; wearing face coverings; and, most important, staying home when sick. The organization discouraged people from gathering in groups or traveling to high-traffic locations and encouraged them to be mindful and respectful of closings intended to curb the spread of disease.[17]

- **COVID-19 Black Lung Working Group:** Encouraging vulnerable individuals to take an active part in protecting their own health and aiding their community's resilience can strengthen the community as a whole. The Center for Appalachian Research in Environmental Sciences, Appalshop, Shaping Our Appalachian Region, Appalachian Citizens' Law Center, and WMMT-FM (a radio station located in Whitesburg, Kentucky) formed a COVID-19 Black Lung Working Group. The group identified a need to educate people in coal-producing counties about the seriousness of COVID-19. The group promoted prevention behaviors, created public service announcements, and helped distribute masks and other resources to current and former coal miners to mitigate exposure to the virus among this high-risk population.[18]

- **Judge executive in Harlan County, Kentucky:** Community members who are regularly involved in one another's lives may be empowered to help their neighbors when disaster strikes. Therefore, building social connectedness can be an important emergency preparedness action. On May 6, 2020, Harlan County, Kentucky, identified its first individual with COVID-19, and the county was prepared. The judge executive in Harlan County had been encouraging residents to protect their community since Kentucky's first case of COVID-19 had been identified exactly two months earlier. The tight-knit groups centered around churches and schools tended to check on one another and share information. He capitalized on this sense of connectedness, addressing the community through various media sources and telling residents, "What we have to remember is that all of us as a member of this county, state, country and world have a responsibility to protect the health of ourselves, the ones that rely on us and look out for each other." He promoted adherence to state and CDC guidelines early in the pandemic, while assuring the community, "We will all get through this together." He also worked with the community to take swift action when COVID-19 cases rose rapidly due to individual complacency and out-of-state travel around the July 4 holiday. The county expanded testing and contact tracing and distributed free face masks. By working with local businesses and capitalizing on community connectedness, the county was able to slow the spread of the virus.[19]

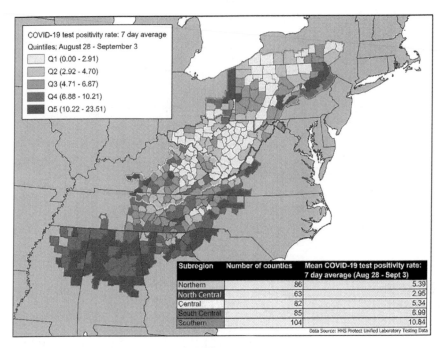

Figure 10.1. Seven-day average COVID-19 test positivity rates by county and subregion in Appalachia (August 28–September 3, 2020).

Early efforts to mitigate the health effects of the virus in Central Appalachia saved lives. Even though the Central subregion has some of the highest prevalence rates of conditions known to increase the risk of severe illness from COVID-19, basic public health measures (e.g., contact tracing, social distancing, mask requirements, stay-at-home orders, and good hand hygiene) managed to contain the spread. Figure 10.1 shows the seven-day average of COVID-19 test positivity rates in Appalachia early in the outbreak (August 28–September 3, 2020). Notably, the Central subregion had the second-lowest rate, while the South Central and Southern subregions had the highest; overall test positivity rates were similar in these subregions (figure 10.2). By September 1, 2020, the Northern, North Central, and Central subregions had met World Health Organization (WHO) criteria for easing some COVID-19–related restrictions by maintaining a 5 percent or lower positivity rate (i.e., percentage of all tests positive for COVID-19) for at least two weeks.[20]

After schools reopened in September 2020, all subregions saw an increase in testing positivity rates, based on a three-day average (figure 10.3). Central Appalachia had fewer cases per 100,000 than all other Appalachian subregions

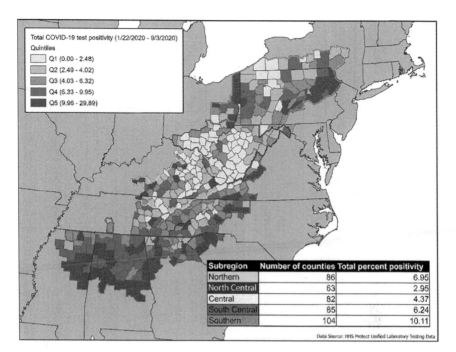

Subregion	Number of counties	Total percent positivity
Northern	86	6.95
North Central	63	2.95
Central	82	4.37
South Central	85	6.24
Southern	104	10.11

Data Source: HHS Protect Unified Laboratory Testing Data

Figure 10.2. Overall average COVID-19 test positivity rates by county and subregion in Appalachia (January 22–September 3, 2020).

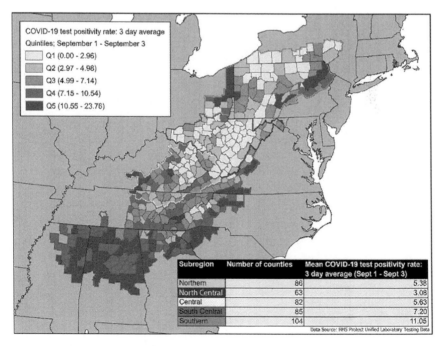

Subregion	Number of counties	Mean COVID-19 test positivity rate: 3 day average (Sept 1 - Sept 3)
Northern	86	5.38
North Central	63	3.08
Central	82	5.63
South Central	85	7.20
Southern	104	11.05

Data Source: HHS Protect Unified Laboratory Testing Data

Figure 10.3. Three-day average COVID-19 test positivity rates by county and subregion in Appalachia (September 1–3, 2020).

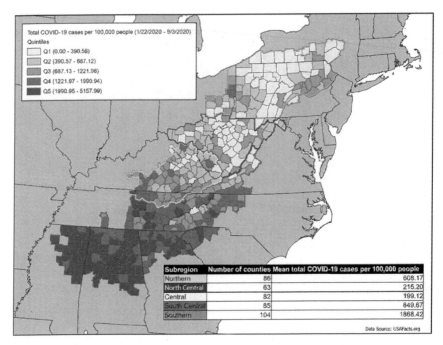

Figure 10.4. Total COVID-19 cases per 100,000 by county and subregion in Appalachia (January 22–September 3, 2020).

(figure 10.4), and the Central and South Central subregions had the lowest case fatality rates, while the Northern and North Central subregions had the highest (figure 10.5). The mean deaths per 100,000 people was highest in Southern Appalachia (figure 10.6). These data align with differences among states containing Appalachian counties during March–July 2020, with initial spikes in cases and excess deaths during the spring surge in the northeastern United States, followed by a summer surge and uncontrolled spread in hot spots throughout the southern United States.[21]

The Kentucky Department for Public Health produced a daily composite state-level COVID-19 status score. It used an indicator monitoring report tool to combine multiple data elements, allowing a systematic assessment of the state's mitigation, response, and reopening efforts. These composites helped guide decision making at the county level. For instance, the Pike County COVID-19 Task Force effectively scaled up mitigation measures to achieve an overall positivity rate of 1.04 percent. Three weeks after the traditional miners' vacation week and the Fourth of July holiday, Pike County experienced its highest weekly positivity rate, at 2.6 percent. Many cases during late July

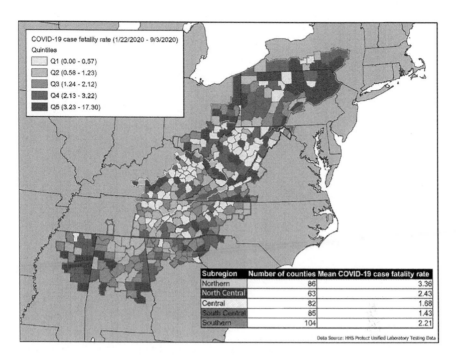

Subregion	Number of counties	Mean COVID-19 case fatality rate
Northern	86	3.36
North Central	63	2.43
Central	82	1.68
South Central	85	1.43
Southern	104	2.21

Data Source: HHS Protect Unified Laboratory Testing Data

Figure 10.5. COVID-19 case fatality rate by county and subregion in Appalachia (January 22–September 3, 2020).

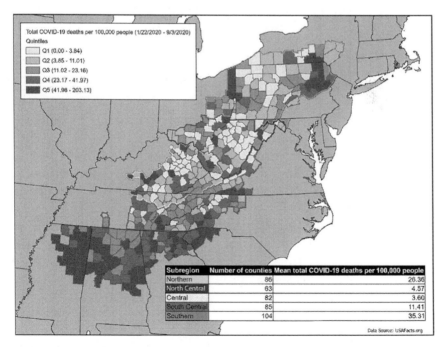

Subregion	Number of counties	Mean total COVID-19 deaths per 100,000 people
Northern	86	26.36
North Central	63	4.57
Central	82	3.60
South Central	85	11.41
Southern	104	35.31

Data Source: USAFacts.org

Figure 10.6. Total COVID-19 deaths per 100,000 by county and subregion in Appalachia (January 22–September 3, 2020).

occurred as families returned from the Carolina beaches and other vacation destinations. As of September 1, 2020, Pike County had reported 319 cases since the start of the pandemic; 25 patients were hospitalized, and 3 had died (0.09 percent mortality rate). Considering the existing health disparities and high prevalence of comorbidities, local public health experts had anticipated a much higher mortality rate in the county.[22]

From March 17 to April 16, 2020, West Virginia saw a rise in COVID-19 cases among residents and staff in nursing homes. Although it was a resource-intensive endeavor, from April 21 to May 8 West Virginia conducted universal testing in all 123 of the state's nursing homes. This proved to be essential for limiting COVID-19 transmission in nursing homes and reducing the pandemic's impact on this high-risk population. In Mingo County, West Virginia, cases were sparsely reported by the local health department, with only 17 by June 30, 2020. However, 130 cases were reported in July; these were largely attributed to residents' vacation travel outside the area and to three significant events—a wedding, a wake, and a church gathering. By August 1, there were a total of 147 cases and 3 deaths in Mingo County, and as of September 1, the county reported an additional 112 cases and 3 deaths. Mingo County continued collaborating with community partners and testing for COVID-19; approximately 4,200 tests were conducted by September 1, with an overall positivity rate of 6.16 percent. Although the county experienced a significant increase in both cases and positivity rate in August, the local health department and community continued to create and implement mitigation strategies and educational initiatives.[23]

As the pandemic extended into October 2020, these local response coalitions continued to prepare and adapt to the ever-evolving informational needs related to the phases of the pandemic. By November 1, nearly all subregions of Appalachia were in an upward trajectory for COVID-19 incidence, similar to the trend seen across North America, Europe, and the eastern Mediterranean region, which coincided with predictions of increased transmission if mitigation measures were relaxed and indoor social gatherings increased as colder weather arrived.[24]

Although public health efforts aimed at prevention remain a challenge in the region, a movement for creating a "culture of health in Appalachia" produced better-than-expected results early in the pandemic, given the region's social determinants and resource limitations. "What you find instead are community members who are committed to creating better opportunities for themselves and their neighbors to live the healthiest lives possible. You find leaders from all walks of life coming together and using the assets they have at hand to build a local 'Culture of Health,'" said Hilary Heishman, program officer at the

Robert Wood Johnson Foundation, who was quoted in a 2018 ARC press release. "While Appalachia lags behind the rest of the nation on many key measures of health, the Appalachian Regional Commission . . . finds that local communities, even with modest resources, can positively influence the health and well-being of their citizens when they share a sense of strength and resiliency," said ARC federal cochair Tim Thomas. Rural areas face resource constraints, so local health departments operating in these communities collectively have to identify and focus on the minimum proficiency needed to respond to emergencies.[25]

Trust for America's Health (TFAH) has pointed out that "the United States must expand efforts to better protect Americans from new infectious disease threats . . . or antibiotic-resistant Superbugs and resurging illnesses like whooping cough, tuberculosis and gonorrhea." According to Jeffrey Levi, executive director of TFAH, "The overuse of antibiotics and underuse of vaccinations along with unstable and insufficient funding have left major gaps in our country's ability to prepare for infectious disease threats." Communities cannot afford to be complacent. Infectious diseases can disrupt the lives of millions of Americans, as seen during the COVID-19 pandemic. These diseases contribute to billions of dollars in excess health care costs each year. Interventions for disease prevention are more likely to succeed with community participation. It is important to consider the distinct, heterogeneous communities in Appalachia that share a strong history and cultural heritage when developing health programs in the region. Public health practitioners in Appalachia are frequently asked to adapt evidence-based programs created for other populations to Appalachian communities; however, attempts to generalize programs tested among specific populations defined by race or ethnicity run the risk of reducing program fidelity. As a federally defined region in the United States, Appalachia may benefit from a regional approach to public health surveillance to support the collection and analysis of health-related data.[26]

Equitable development and a revamping of aging systems are required to allow easier access to health care. Improving partnerships among clinicians, researchers, government, and industry to detect and diagnose disease, conduct research, develop effective countermeasures to prevent and treat disease, and deliver these therapies effectively to those who need them is essential. Clinicians are often the first to encounter cases of emerging infectious diseases, and they need to work closely with local health departments to quickly identify and respond to outbreaks. Rural health care providers, in particular, benefit from flexibility in the delivery of health care, such as eliminating regulatory burdens that limit the availability of clinical professionals and hinder continuity of care for their patients. Improving the accessibility of high-quality telehealth services and implementing reporting, staffing, and supervision flexibility for providers are important considerations to meet the needs of rural Appalachians.

Limited transportation options and hospital closures have also created barriers to care in rural communities. In Appalachia, many patients must plan well in advance to arrange transportation for long-distance travel to receive basic care, and there are long wait times and transportation challenges for specialty care as well. When the COVID-19 pandemic struck, this challenge was intensified as state shutdown orders kept many patients in their homes. Within weeks, COVID-19 had transformed health care, leading to an unprecedented rise in the use of telehealth services. To respond to the urgent need to protect Medicare beneficiaries from the dangers of COVID-19, Congress included telehealth provisions in the Coronavirus Aid, Relief, and Economic Security (CARES) Act.[27] On March 13, 2020, President Trump made an emergency declaration under the Stafford Act and the National Emergencies Act, empowering the Centers for Medicare & Medicaid Services (CMS) to issue waivers that allowed Medicare beneficiaries to receive telehealth services in any location, including their homes, and to expand the scope of these services, making it easier for different types of health care providers to offer a wider range of telehealth services. CMS observed an immediate, dramatic increase in the use of telehealth services, and by April 2020, soon after the pandemic hit the United States, nearly half (43.5 percent) of Medicare recipients' primary care visits were provided through telehealth, compared with less than 1 percent (0.1 percent) in February. According to public health leaders in rural areas, the Appalachian region could capitalize on these changes in telehealth established during the COVID-19 pandemic to improve access to health care in the future. There is broad interest in making pandemic-related telehealth flexibilities permanent and access more equitable. Small towns are becoming "innovation hubs" in rural areas out of necessity, working in a multisector model to come up with creative solutions to problems, such as turning a distillery into a hand-sanitizer production site for local hospitals. It could be worthwhile to package these ideas as best practices, disseminate them more broadly, and share the innovations and leadership happening in the Appalachian region.[28]

To prevent the next pandemic, Dr. Ali Khan, former director of the CDC's Center for Preparedness and Response, emphasizes that a comprehensive approach is warranted—one that focuses not only on the microbe but also on the role of communities and individuals in creating the circumstances that give rise to these events. Weather events, microbes, and man-made disasters continue to challenge community leaders charged with keeping residents safe.

Supporting public health systems at the local level will be beneficial in the face of future public health crises, as systems ramp up their infrastructure to address them. Even with the latest scientific guidance and expertise at the international, national, and state levels, public health happens locally in every community. By building better public health systems, communities and individuals can become more engaged with the concept of personal preparedness.[29]

To decrease excessive loss of life from pandemics and other public health emergencies, communities can implement innovative evidence-based programs to address regional disparities in health care access, quality of care, and health outcomes. There is a need for trained public health professionals who can translate hardships faced in the midst of a response into specific public health actions. County planning should include a consideration of environmental and public health policies. By strengthening community partnerships and collaborations, the region can focus on improved community health and disease prevention. Appalachia's commitment at all levels of community preparedness will ensure that it continues to overcome public health emergencies. Through the identification of new opportunities and a regional and strategic approach to achieving results, hope, and resiliency, it stands ready for the next challenge.[30]

Notes

The findings and conclusions of this chapter are those of the authors and do not necessarily represent the official position of the Centers for Disease Control and Prevention. We gratefully acknowledge the contributions of Ari Whiteman, PhD, MSc (Geospatial Research, Analysis, and Services Program, CDC), for accessing data sets to create the county-level maps of Appalachia; Tal Jones (Shaping Our Appalachian Region) for a thoughtful review of the chapter; Jack Colbert, MLIS (Stephen B. Thacker Library, CDC), for an in-depth literature review and research; and Robyn Sobelson, PhD (Center for State, Tribal, Local, and Territorial Support, CDC), for her thoughtful review, patience, counsel, and unwavering positivity during CDC clearance.

1. Adrian K. Ong and David L. Heymann, "Microbes and Humans: The Long Dance," *Bulletin of the World Health Organization* 85, no. 6 (2007): 422; David L. Heymann, "Emerging and Other Infectious Diseases: Epidemiology and Control," *World Health Statistics Quarterly* 50, no. 3–4 (1997): 158–60.

2. National Governors' Association, *Comprehensive Emergency Management: A Governor's Guide* (Washington, DC: Center for Policy Research, 1979), 64; Kathleen J. Tierney, Michael K. Lindell, and Ronald W. Perry, eds., *Facing the Unexpected: Disaster Preparedness and Response in the United States* (Washington, DC: Joseph Henry Press, 2001), 320; *All Disasters Are Local—So Are Many Resources* (Washington, DC: FEMA, 2020), https://www.fema.gov/media-library-data/1383655930102-a46a0f5a70ac8fece4cd30ebe8ae89fe/Regionalization.pdf; CDC, "Center for Preparedness and Response: State and Local Readiness," reviewed July 16, 2020, https://www.cdc.gov/cpr/whatwedo/phep.htm; Jeffrey

Howard, "Fiscal Challenges and Anticipated Changes to Kentucky's Population Health System," *Journal of Appalachian Health* 2, no. 3 (2020): 1–4.

3. Jeanne S. Ringel et al., *Lessons Learned from the State and Local Public Health Response to Hurricane Katrina*, RAND Working Paper prepared for the US Department of Health and Human Services (Washington, DC: Gulf States Policy Institute and RAND Health, 2007); Jonathan M. Links et al., "COPEWELL: A Conceptual Framework and System Dynamics Model for Predicting Community Functioning and Resilience after Disasters," *Disaster Medicine and Public Health Preparedness* 12, no. 1 (2018): 127–37; Margaret A. Riggs et al., "Resident Cleanup Activities, Characteristics of Flood-Damaged Homes and Airborne Microbial Concentrations in New Orleans, Louisiana, October 2005," *Environmental Research* 106, no. 3 (2008): 401–9; Kristin J. Cummings et al., "Respirator Donning in Post-Hurricane New Orleans," *Emerging Infectious Diseases* 13, no. 5 (2007): 700–707.

4. S. K. Mishra, "Hospital Overcrowding," *Western Journal of Medicine* 174, no. 3 (2001): 170; Links et al., "COPEWELL"; Jennifer Schroeder and Erin D. Bouldin, "Inclusive Public Health Preparedness Program to Promote Resilience in Rural Appalachia (2016–2018)," *American Journal of Public Health* 109, suppl. 4 (2019): S283–85.

5. Eugene J. Lengerich et al., "Images of Appalachia," *Preventing Chronic Disease* 3, no. 4 (2006): A112; Kelvin Pollard and Linda A. Jacobsen, *The Appalachian Region: A Data Overview from the 2014–2018 American Community Survey* (Washington, DC: ARC, 2020), 180; ESRI, "A Story Map: Appalachian Mountains," https://www.arcgis.com/apps/MapJournal/index.html?appid=2c4e728395b44d2cbc70d761adb14d1d; Linda H. Banks et al., "Disaster Impact on Impoverished Area of US: An Inter-Professional Mixed Method Study," *Prehospital and Disaster Medicine* 31, no. 6 (2016): 583–92.

6. Rebecca Reynolds Yonker and Ben Tobin, "Rockslide Causes Fiery Train Crash in Kentucky, Sends Rail Cars into River," *Louisville Courier-Journal*, February 13, 2020, https://www.courier-journal.com/story/news/local/2020/02/13/csx-train-derails-kentucky-after-rockslide/4747750002/; Roberto G. Lucchini et al., "A Comparative Assessment of Major International Disasters: The Need for Exposure Assessment, Systematic Emergency Preparedness, and Lifetime Health Care," *BMC Public Health* 17, no. 1 (2017): 46.

7. Qun Li et al., "Early Transmission Dynamics in Wuhan, China, of Novel Coronavirus-Infected Pneumonia," *New England Journal of Medicine* 382, no. 13 (2020): 1199–207; Yosra A. Helmy et al., "The COVID-19 Pandemic: A Comprehensive Review of Taxonomy, Genetics, Epidemiology, Diagnosis, Treatment and Control," *Journal of Clinical Medicine* 9, no. 4 (2020): 1225; CDC, "COVID-19 & IPC Overview," updated August 12, 2020, https://www.cdc.gov/coronavirus/2019-ncov/hcp/non-us-settings/overview/index.html#background; Lauren M. Oppizzi and Susan Speraw, "Federal Emergency Management Agency Response in Rural Appalachia: A Tale of Miscommunication, Unrealistic Expectations, and 'Hurt, Hurt, Hurt,'" *Nursing Clinics of North America* 51, no. 4 (2016): 599–611; Brystana G. Kaufman, Rebecca Whitaker, George Pink, and G. Mark Holmes, "Half of Rural Residents at High Risk of Serious Illness Due to COVID-19, Creating Stress on Rural Hospitals," *Journal of Rural Health* 00 (2020): 1–7; Banks et al., "Disaster Impact."

8. Chris Kenning, "Once Seemingly Insulated, Kentucky's Appalachian Counties Scramble to Stop COVID-19 Outbreak," *Louisville Courier-Journal*, July 31, 2020, https://www.courier-journal.com/story/news/local/2020/07/31/covid-19-appalachia-tiny-health-departments-struggle-outbreak/5526869002/; Tammy Riley, director, Pike County (KY) Health Department, personal communication with author (Riggs), 2020; Keith Blankenship, director, Mingo County (WV) Health Department, personal communication with author (Riggs), 2020.

9. Peter Ranscombe, "Rural Areas at Risk during COVID-19 Pandemic," *Lancet Infectious Diseases* 20, no. 5 (2020): 545; ARC, "County Economic Status in Appalachia, FY 2021," https://www.arc.gov/map/county-economic-status-in-appalachia-fy-2021/; Darshana T. Shah, "The COVID-19 Crisis: How Rural Appalachia Is Handling the Pandemic," *Marshall Journal of Medicine* 6, no. 2 (2020): 1.

10. CDC, "Coronavirus Disease 2019 (COVID-19): Older Adults," updated September 11, 2020, https://www.cdc.gov/coronavirus/2019-ncov/need-extra-precautions/older-adults .html; Pollard and Jacobsen, *Appalachian Region*; CDC, "Coronavirus Disease 2019 (COVID-19): People with Certain Medical Conditions," updated November 2, 2020, https://www.cdc .gov/coronavirus/2019-ncov/need-extra-precautions/people-with-medical-conditions .html; CDC, "Overweight & Obesity: Adult Obesity Facts," reviewed June 29, 2020, https:// www.cdc.gov/obesity/data/adult.html; Hilda Razzaghi et al., "Estimated County-Level Prevalence of Selected Underlying Medical Conditions Associated with Increased Risk for Severe COVID-19 Illness—United States, 2018," *Morbidity and Mortality Weekly Report* 69, no. 29 (2020): 945–50.

11. Angel N. Desai and Payal Patel, "Stopping the Spread of COVID-19," *JAMA* 323, no. 15 (2020): 1516; John T. Brooks, Jay C. Butler, and Robert R. Redfield, "Universal Masking to Prevent SARS-CoV-2 Transmission—The Time Is Now," *JAMA* 324, no. 7 (2020): 635–37; M. Joshua Hendrix, Charles Walde, Kendra Findley, and Robin Trotman, "Absence of Apparent Transmission of SARS-CoV-2 from Two Stylists after Exposure at a Hair Salon with a Universal Face Covering Policy—Springfield, Missouri, May 2020," *Morbidity and Mortality Weekly Report* 69, no. 28 (2020): 930–32; Riley, personal communication; Blankenship, personal communication.

12. Jennifer R. Davis et al., "The Impact of Disasters on Populations with Health and Health Care Disparities," *Disaster Medicine and Public Health Preparedness* 4, no. 1 (2010): 30–38; Bruce Behringer and Gilbert H. Friedell, "Appalachia: Where Place Matters in Health," *Preventing Chronic Disease* 3, no. 4 (2006): A113; Earl S. Ford et al., "Chronic Disease in Health Emergencies: In the Eye of the Hurricane," *Preventing Chronic Disease* 3, no. 2 (2006): A46; ARC, Foundation for a Healthy Kentucky, and RWJF, "Creating a Culture of Health in Appalachia: Disparities and Bright Spots," 2020, https://healthinappalachia.org/.

13. Brian Martin et al., "Qualitative Study of Public Health Preparedness and Response to the Rabid Raccoon Discovered in Wise County, Virginia," *Journal of Veterinary Medicine* (2019): 1–5, article no. 5734590.

14. Jill Crainshaw, "Dusty Shoes: Appalachia Wisdom Fertilizing the Future of Religious Leadership," *Journal of Appalachian Health* 1, no. 1 (2019): 34–39; Behringer and Friedell, "Appalachia"; Stephen M. Petrany, Deb Koester, and Robert Walker, "Reflections on West Virginia's Early COVID-19 Experience," *Marshall Journal of Medicine* 6, no. 2 (2020): 20–21; David B. Resnik, "Scientific Research and the Public Trust," *Science and Engineering Ethics* 17, no. 3 (2011): 399–409; Oppizzi and Speraw, "Federal Emergency Management Agency Response."

15. Public Health Emergency, "Community Resilience," reviewed June 9, 2015, https:// www.phe.gov/Preparedness/planning/abc/Pages/community-resilience.aspx#:~:text =Individual%20health%20and%20resilience%20is,People%20should%20try%20to%3 A&text=Engage%20in%20community%20or%20neighborhood%20preparedness%20 activities; Links et al., "COPEWELL."

16. Tauna Gulley et al., "The Health Wagon Partners with the Virginia Department of Health to Provide COVID-19 Testing in Rural Southwest Virginia," *Journal of Appalachian Health* 2, no. 3 (2020): 146–49.

17. Active Southern West Virginia, "Kids Run Club—Virtual Edition," *Active SWV Blog*, 2020, https://activeswv.org/kids-run-club-virtual-edition/.

18. University of Kentucky College of Medicine, "UK-CARES: Recommendations for Those with Black Lung Disease," 2020, https://ukcares.med.uky.edu/black-lung-disease.

19. Emily Sargent, "Mosley Addresses COVID-19 Panic, Precautions," *Harlan Enterprise*, March 17, 2020, https://www.harlanenterprise.net/2020/03/17/mosley-addresses-covid-19-panic-precautions/; Dan Mosley, judge executive, Harlan County, KY, personal communication with author (Riggs), 2020.

20. WHO, "Public Health Criteria to Adjust Public Health and Social Measures in the Context of COVID-19," 2020, https://apps.who.int/iris/handle/10665/332073.

21. Alexandra M. Oster et al., "Trends in Number and Distribution of COVID-19 Hotspot Counties—United States, March 8–July 15, 2020," *Morbidity and Mortality Weekly Report* 69, no. 33 (2020): 1127–32; Howard Bauchner and Phil B. Fontanarosa, "Excess Deaths and the Great Pandemic of 2020," *JAMA* 324, no. 15 (2020): 1504–5; Steven H. Woolf, "Excess Deaths from COVID-19 and Other Causes, March–July 2020," *JAMA* 324, no. 15 (2020): 1562–64.

22. Kate Varela et al., "Primary Indicators to Systematically Monitor COVID-19 Mitigation and Response—Kentucky, May 19–July 15, 2020," *Morbidity and Mortality Weekly Report* 69, no. 34 (2020): 1173–76; Riley, personal communication.

23. Shannon M. McBee et al., "Notes from the Field: Universal Statewide Laboratory Testing for SARS-CoV-2 in Nursing Homes—West Virginia, April 21–May 8, 2020," *Morbidity and Mortality Weekly Report* 69, no. 34 (2020): 1177–79; Blankenship, personal communication.

24. CDC, "COVIDView," https://www.cdc.gov/coronavirus/2019-ncov/covid-data/covidview/index.html; WHO, "Weekly Epidemiological Update," October 27, 2020, https://www.who.int/publications/m/item/weekly-epidemiological-update-27-october-2020; Cory Merow and Mark C. Urban, "Seasonality and Uncertainty in Global COVID-19 Growth Rates," *Proceedings of the National Academy of Sciences of the United States* 117, no. 44 (2020): 27456–64.

25. ARC et al., "Creating a Culture of Health in Appalachia"; Wendy Wasserman, "New Research and Website Highlight Health in Appalachia," ARC, July 24, 2018, https://www.arc.gov/news/www-healthy-ky-org/; Scott Santibañez et al., "Strengthening Rural States' Capacity to Prepare for and Respond to Emerging Infectious Diseases, 2013–2015," *Southern Medical Journal* 112, no. 2 (2019): 101–5.

26. Trust for America's Health, "Outbreaks: Protecting Americans from Infectious Diseases," December 18, 2014, https://www.tfah.org/releases/outbreaks2014/; Lengerich et al., "Images of Appalachia."

27. Anthony S. Fauci, "Emerging and Reemerging Infectious Diseases: The Perpetual Challenge," *Academic Medicine* 80, no. 12 (2005): 1079–85; Santibañez et al., "Strengthening Rural States' Capacity"; Executive Order 13941, *Weekly Compilation of Presidential Documents* (August 6, 2020); Health Resources and Services Administration, "Rural Hospital Programs," reviewed November 2020, https://www.hrsa.gov/rural-health/rural-hospitals; Brook Calton, Nauzley Abedini, and Michael Fratkin, "Telemedicine in the Time of Coronavirus," *Journal of Pain and Symptom Management* 60, no. 1 (2020): e12–14; Arielle Bosworth et al., *Issue Brief: Medicare Beneficiary Use of Telehealth Visits: Early Data from the Start of the COVID-19 Pandemic* (Washington, DC: ASPE, 2020), https://aspe.hhs.gov/system/files/pdf/263866/HP_IssueBrief_MedicareTelehealth_final7.29.20.pdf; Coronavirus Aid, Relief, and Economic Security Act of 2020, Pub. L. No. 116–136, 134 Stat. 281 (2020).

28. Executive Order 13941; US Department of Health and Human Services, "HHS Issues New Report Highlighting Dramatic Trends in Medicare Beneficiary Telehealth Utilization amid COVID-19," July 28, 2020, https://www.hhs.gov/about/news/2020/07/28/hhs-issues-new-report-highlighting-dramatic-trends-in-medicare-beneficiary-telehealth-utilization-amid-covid-19.html; Alfredo Morabia with Shauntice Allen, Wendy Braund, Michael Meit, and Eduardo Sanchez, "Should Public Health Lean on Rural America to Revamp Itself," August 20, 2020, produced by the *American Journal of Public Health*, MP3 audio, https://soundcloud.com/alfredomorabia/ajph-september-2020-should-public-health-lean-on-rural-america-to-revamp-itself-english; Bosworth et al., *Issue Brief: Medicare Beneficiary Use of Telehealth;* Calton, Abedini, and Fratkin, "Telemedicine."

29. Ali S. Khan, *The Next Pandemic: On the Front Lines against Humankind's Gravest Dangers* (New York: PublicAffairs, 2016).

30. Margaret A. Riggs, "Ice Storm 2009: Kentucky's Epidemiological Response," *Domestic Preparedness Journal*, June 3, 2009, https://www.domprep.com/healthcare/ice-storm-2009-kentuckys-regional-response/.

11

Conclusion

RANDY WYKOFF, F. DOUGLAS SCUTCHFIELD,
RON R. ROACH, AND RON ELLER

Appalachia, like many other parts of the United States, is a complex region.
Defined at various times by its geology, geography, history, culture, socioeconomic conditions, politics, and other factors, it is a diverse place shaped by the
larger society around it. The people of Appalachia, however they are defined,
have some of the worst health statistics of any group of people in the United
States. Whether one looks at health behaviors (e.g., smoking, opioid misuse)
or health outcomes (e.g., life expectancy, rates of heart disease), the people of
Appalachia are less healthy than the rest of America and, in fact, less healthy
than the people who live in the non-Appalachian counties of the same states.

As described in this book, there are many reasons why Appalachian individuals' health status lags behind that of the rest of the nation and why health
disparities within Appalachia are severe in some subregions (Central Appalachia in particular). These reasons include environmental influences (the workplace environment as well as the ambient environment), socioeconomic factors,
cultural issues, health behaviors, and access to services, among others. When
examined independently, many of these factors seem to be improving in Appalachia. Over the past few decades, for example, smoking rates in the region have
declined. Over the same period, the number of counties identified as economically distressed has also declined. Educational attainment has increased, as more
Appalachians are graduating from high school than ever before. Geographic
isolation—impacted first by railroads for the coal industry, roads and highways,
military service, television, and, most recently, the internet—has steadily been
reduced.

Yet despite these apparent improvements, the health of the people of
Appalachia still lags behind the health of the rest of the country in several
important areas. This seeming contradiction is explained, in part, by two facts.
The first is that while many of the factors that impact health are improving in
Appalachia, they are improving more slowly there than in the rest of the country. For example, smoking rates are going down in Appalachia, but they are
decreasing more slowly than elsewhere in America. Although there are fewer
economically distressed counties in Appalachia than there were a few decades

ago, many areas of rural and Central Appalachia continue to be severely distressed. Moreover, throughout the United States there has been a growing divide between the wealthiest Americans and the poorest Americans. Today, the gap between the income of the top fifth and bottom fifth of Americans is more than 50 percent wider than it was sixty years ago.[1]

The second factor that explains the apparent contradiction is that new health challenges have arisen in the region to counterbalance the improvements made. These challenges—including opioid misuse, suicide, social isolation, and the environmental impact of surface mining—have disproportionately affected the people of Appalachia. Like residents of other highland regions, individuals in Appalachia face mixed prospects as a result of these challenges. On the one hand, the region has tremendous assets on which to build: incredible natural resources and beauty, a rich culture and history, and resilient, hardworking residents. On the other hand, the region is still trying to overcome decades of marginalization, stigmatization, and economic exploitation. In addition to socioeconomic and demographic factors, the cultural landscape of Appalachia is undeniably different than it was even twenty-five years ago. This change is partly a reflection of Appalachia's connection to four larger national and global shifts during that period: (1) increased economic globalization, with the proliferation of free-trade agreements, trade imbalances, regional economic declines, and rising income gaps; (2) shifting demographic patterns, with greater immigration and increased diversity; (3) rapid technological changes, including the internet, social media, and industrial mechanization; and (4) environmental challenges, the shift to more sustainable energy sources, and the growing threat of climate change.

But the region has seen radical change before. In the spring of 1919, mere months before John C. Campbell's untimely death, he and Olive returned to northeastern Tennessee, where they had begun their original survey of the southern mountains just ten years earlier. They were amazed at the changes that had taken place in such a short time. In nearby Johnson City, they marveled at the population growth and the new railroads serving the area. As they left the train in Erwin and traveled into rural Unicoi County, they were struck by a newly opened pottery factory and silk mill, paved roads, modern bridges, automobiles, rural telephones, and corresponding changes in the way of life. This experience led Campbell to reflect on the region:

> The country was indeed a strange mingling of new and old, whose contrasts were not less striking in that once remote part of the mountains where at last we reached our destination. As in our national capital the young and prosperous lived side by side with the old and humble; the

modern was close to the pioneer. . . . The Highland country is in truth a land of paradoxes and contradictions, because here in a restricted area are taking place all the changes that are going on in the world elsewhere.[2]

This is even truer today: more than ever, Appalachia is connected to and reflects global forces. As we begin the third decade of the twenty-first century, humanity may be living through the most rapid transformations in its long history. We also face incredible challenges to peace, security, health, quality of life, and the very survival of the planet. The increasing globalization of the world means that—whether we live in the Alps, the Himalayas, the Appalachians, or elsewhere—we will face these challenges together.

Given these new challenges, people in the world's mountain regions now realize how much they have in common and how important their regions are globally. Ironically, with the prevailing marginalization and resource extraction habitually brought to bear on the mountains, people worldwide are recognizing that how we deal with problems in the highlands can have far-reaching consequences for the lowlands. As Sternberg opines: "We are all part of our world, and what we do in the spaces around us not only shapes them but shapes ourselves. We can create places that devour and destroy the environment and that in turn destroy us. Or we can do the opposite—create places that help us to live in harmony with the environment and sustain our health." If we can find a solution in Appalachia to the problems of transitioning to a more sustainable way of living—economically, environmentally, and socially— the same solutions can be applied elsewhere.[3]

Ultimately, the overarching question is whether Appalachia can break out of the educational and economic inequalities contributing to its long-term health challenges. These challenges are complex and intertwined. Take income, for example: We know that children in the United States born to parents living in the bottom economic quintile are ten times more likely to remain in the bottom quintile than they are to reach the top quintile. The rich stay rich, and the poor stay poor. Combined with the widening income gap between the richest and poorest Americans, this trend means that regions where there are more poor people—across America, but more specifically in Appalachia—will continue to see widening gaps compared with regions where there are more wealthy people. Because poverty is so tightly interwoven with health, regions like Appalachia can expect to see greater health disparities than wealthier regions, as health disparities mirror economic gaps.[4]

Educational divides intensify regional health challenges in a similar fashion. For example, we know that the educational level of parents has a tremendous impact on their children's level of educational achievement. This means that, over time, there will be a widening gap in educational achievement between those parts of the country where parents have more education and those parts where parents have less education. Because education is tightly interwoven with income, and because both education and income are related to health, regions like Appalachia—where parents have, on average, received less education than parents in other regions—can expect to see widening health gaps compared with more educated parts of the country. Unless the region can break this cycle, the health gap will continue to widen for the foreseeable future.[5]

In addition to economic and educational divides, health behaviors contribute to the patterns observed in Appalachia. Studies have shown that children of parents who smoke are more likely to become smokers themselves. Similarly, children of obese parents are more likely to be obese. The difficulty of reversing cultural trends in health behaviors has far-reaching implications for the health status of the entire region. We know that sedentary lifestyle, obesity, and smoking are more common in areas with higher rates of poverty, so children living in poverty are more likely to adopt a range of less healthy behaviors. Research has shown that there are ways to intervene in these "intergenerational" cycles, but little research has addressed these complex factors in rural Appalachia.[6]

As this complex mix of poverty, lack of education, and poor health behaviors continues to exert an intergenerational impact on health, it becomes clear that, in the absence of major social changes, these cycles will continue. Thus, Appalachians will likely become increasingly less healthy than folks in the rest of the country. What these necessary changes will be, and whether the journey toward them will be easy or difficult, remains unknown. Regardless of this uncertainty, this book has provided some suggestions for those who are committed to the mountains of Appalachia.

Data on the health and welfare of Appalachia are necessary to track changes—both positive and negative—in the region. In many cases, the data already exist (e.g., the Behavioral Risk Factor Survey) but are not analyzed specifically for Appalachia. Official reports and compilations by states and counties in Appalachia should be made available as databases for those who live and work in the region to increase understanding and identify potential targets for improving Appalachian health and welfare. Where specific data do not exist, provisions should be made to collect and report such data for those committed to the health of the region.

Similarly, there are evidence-based interventions for many of the ills afflicting Appalachia; however, many health policy and behavioral interventions have not been developed specifically for Appalachia. Although evidence-driven interventions to address health behavior may exist and should be implemented, it is imperative to recognize that specific interventions drawn from other areas may or may not work in an Appalachia community, given the character of the region and its people. To increase the chances of success, interventions need to be developed specifically for Appalachian communities.

Future research should account for the myriad sociocultural factors that constrain access to health care in the mountains. Further, it should acknowledge the complex lived experiences of Appalachia's people as they navigate both the health care system and challenges to their own well-being. What works with research subjects in San Diego will not necessarily work in Perry County, Kentucky, as these landscapes differ tremendously.

Ideally, interventions should be tailored to the specific setting, but findings from Appalachian research can, in some cases, be generalized to other settings. Investigations into issues of concern in Appalachia may shed light on those issues elsewhere in the United States; for example, the underlying etiology of substance abuse remains constant, even with changes in the particular drug abused. Moreover, the environment, both ambient and built, affects disease patterns both within Appalachia (e.g., the health impacts of mountaintop removal mining) and outside of it. Issues fraught with political implications must eventually be addressed and any damage remediated.

There are, of course, broader policy issues that must be considered—again, not necessarily unique to Appalachia but certainly applicable to it. Will new and innovative sources of income enable the people of Appalachia to obtain meaningful and productive jobs without leaving the region? Will new approaches ensure that children in Appalachia achieve the same level of education as children in wealthier and more educated parts of the country? Will poor health behaviors become less common in the region? The answers can be found in the efforts of those committed to building a better future for the people of this iconic region and for all Americans, as some solutions may require a substantial change in national policy. One problem with the socioecological determinants of health is the fact that it is difficult to move money across sectors to address the underlying problems of a region. This imbalance is difficult to address by the health sector alone and requires major fundamental changes in the allocation of funds to various sectors, such as health, education, and housing. The necessary and appropriate mechanisms for this allocation and how to address deficiencies are beyond the scope of this book, but these are the fundamental issues that must be addressed if Appalachians, or any other similarly situated poor and unhealthy population, are not to remain poor and sick. As a colleague once remarked, "Am I sick because I am poor or poor because I am sick? It is both; it should be neither."

Notes

1. James Florence et al., "The Depth of Rural Health Disparities in America: ABCDE's," in *Rural Populations and Health: Determinants, Disparities, and Solutions*, ed. Richard A. Crosby, Monica L. Wendel, Robin C. Vanderpool, and Baretta R. Casey (San Francisco: Jossey-Bass, 2012), 51–72; Randolph F. Wykoff, "Tennessee Health Update" (presentation to the Senate Health and Welfare Committee, Washington, DC, January 29, 2020), http://tnga .granicus.com/MediaPlayer.php?view_id=436&clip_id=21370&meta_id=455822 (at 40:00 minute mark).

2. John C. Campbell, *The Southern Highlander and His Homeland* (New York: Russell Sage, 1921), 325–28.

3. Bernard Debarbieux and Martin F. Price, "Mountain Regions: A Global Common Good?" *Mountain Research and Development* 32 (2012): S7–11; Tyson L. Swetnam et al., "Topographically Driven Differences in Energy and Water Constrain Climatic Control on Forest Carbon Sequestration," *Ecosphere* 8, no. 4 (2017): 1–17, https://esajournals .onlinelibrary.wiley.com/doi/epdf/10.1002/ecs2.1797; Hanspeter Liniger and Rolf Weing-artner, "Mountains and Freshwater Supply," *Unasylva* 49, no. 4 (1998), http://www.fao .org/3/w9300e/w9300e08.htm; Esther M. Sternberg, *Healing Places: The Science of Place and Well-being* (Cambridge, MA: Harvard University Press, 2009), 1–2, 10, 291.

4. Randolph F. Wykoff and Olivia Egen, "The Future of Appalachia: Health," *Now and Then Magazine*, https://www.etsu.edu/cph/documents/newsevents/nt_wykoff_012517.pdf; Pew Charitable Trusts, *Pursuing the American Dream: Economic Mobility across Generations* (Washington, DC: Pew Charitable Trusts, 2012), https://www.pewtrusts.org/~/media/legacy /uploadedfiles/wwwpewtrustsorg/reports/economic_mobility/pursuingamericandreampdf .pdf; Olivia Egen et al., "The Health and Social Conditions of the Poorest versus Wealthiest Counties in the United States," *American Journal of Public Health* 107, no. 1 (2017): 130–35; Nancy Adler et al., *Reaching for a Healthier Life: Facts on Socioeconomic Status and Health in the U.S.* (Chicago: John D. and Catherine T. MacArthur Foundation, 2007), https://scholar .harvard.edu/files/davidrwilliams/files/reaching_for_a_healthier_life_0.pdf.

5. RWJF Commission to Build a Healthier America, "Education Matters for Health," RWJF Issue Brief 6, September 2009; Christopher R. Tamborini, ChangHwan Kim, and Arthur Sakamoto, "Education and Lifetime Earnings in the United States," *Demography* 52, no. 4 (2015): 1383–407; Center on Society and Health, "Issue Brief: Why Education Matters to Health: Exploring the Causes," Virginia Commonwealth University, February 13, 2015.

6. Darren Mays et al., "Parental Smoking Exposure and Adolescent Smoking Trajecto-ries," *Pediatrics* 133, no. 6 (2014): 983–91; Robert C. Whitaker et al., "Predicting Obesity in Young Adulthood from Childhood and Parental Obesity" *New England Journal of Medicine* 337 (1997): 869–73; Adler et al., *Reaching for a Healthier Life.*

Acknowledgments

We owe debts of gratitude to a variety of folks. We obviously want to thank our colleagues at the University Press of Kentucky, where Natalie O'Neal Clausen was the acquisitions editor for our work and director Ashley Runyon was supportive of not only this book but also the series focused on underserved populations in the United States. We also want to recognize our colleagues at the University of Kentucky and East Tennessee State University who contributed to the book. In both cases we have colleagues who are knowledgeable about Appalachia and are actively working to improve the health of the region. We took advantage of these two academic institutions, which are committed to serving and supporting health and healing in Appalachia; both the universities and their colleges were key to the successful completion of the book.

The preparation of a book is a difficult and time-consuming task, and the work involves a great deal of attention to detail to comply with the requirements of the press, assure the book's easy flow and readability, and impose consistency across chapters. Rachel Dixon, our fearless editorial assistant, was invaluable in this regard. Her editing and organizing skills are nothing short of miraculous, and for that, we owe her a great deal. She ensured that the book is as good as we could make it.

We also owe a debt of thanks to our families, who gave up nights and weekends with us as we completed the book. They sacrificed so that we might bring this work to you. Their patience and support made the creation of *Appalachian Health* a lot easier than it could have been. We dedicate this work to our families, and Dr. Scutchfield specifically dedicates his work to his grandchildren, Cassandra and Ethan.

F. Douglas Scutchfield
Randy Wykoff

Contributors

Kate Beatty, PhD, MPH

Dr. Kate Beatty is an associate professor in the Department of Health Services Management and Policy at East Tennessee State University's College of Public Health. She is the interim research director of the Center for Rural Health Research in the College of Public Health and is the principal investigator in a multiyear study on the clinical characteristics and practices of contraception access and utilization. Beatty has more than ten years' experience researching rural health issues, including access to public health and health care services, health disparities, and social determinants of health. She is a mixed-methods health services researcher who has led projects on clinical capacities and organizational change and has studied patterns of clinical service delivery in rural and urban health departments, organizational barriers to and facilitators of access to clinical and preventive services, collaboration between local health departments and hospitals, and the role of interorganizational partnerships in the provision of health services in rural communities.

Kelly D. Blake, ScD

Dr. Kelly Blake is a health scientist and program director in the National Cancer Institute's Health Communication and Informatics Research Branch. She also serves as director of NCI's Health Information National Trends Survey (HINTS) and conducts research into how media exposure influences health behavior and attitudes toward public health policy and how communication inequalities and knowledge gaps exacerbate health disparities among disadvantaged populations. Before rejoining NCI in 2009, Blake was a cancer prevention fellow and research assistant at the Dana-Farber Cancer Institute in Boston (2005–2009), as well as a teaching fellow at the Harvard School of Public Health and Kennedy School of Government. Prior to that, she served as a science writer and editor at the Division of Cancer Control and Population Science (2001–2005), a hospital-based public health educator and site coordinator for the West Virginia Rural Health Education Partnerships Program (1997–2001), and a health communication research fellow at the National Institute for Occupational Safety and Health (1996–1997).

Bill Brooks, DrPH, MPH

Dr. Bill Brooks is an assistant professor of biostatistics in the Department of Biostatistics and Epidemiology at East Tennessee State University. He is also an active member of the ETSU Addiction Science Center. His research interests and experience focus on harm reduction and the prevention of accidental overdose among injection drug users. Brooks has been working with community-based organizations in South Central Appalachia since 2010 and has developed many relationships that help keep him apprised of health issues in the region.

Angela L. Carman, DrPH, MBA

Dr. Angela Carman is an assistant professor at the University of Kentucky College of Public Health and a public health management consultant to local health departments and hospitals. A native Kentuckian, she has provided guidance on community health assessments, community health improvement planning, quality improvement training, and strategic planning to more than forty counties in the state. Carman's research focuses on the practice of public health and includes community engagement, public health accreditation readiness, quality improvement, and evidence-based practice implementation. She received specialized training at the Training Institute for Dissemination and Implementation Research in Cancer through the National Cancer Institute in 2018. She is also certified as a human resources professional by the Society for Human Resource Management, as a healthcare executive by the American College of Healthcare Executives, and as a quality improvement associate by the American Society for Quality.

Rachel E. Dixon, MPhil

Rachel Dixon is a recent graduate of the University of Oxford, earning a degree in comparative social policy with concentrations in health policy and the economics of social policy. She formerly served as a resident researcher at the Charles F. Kettering Foundation in Dayton, Ohio. She is the founder and CEO of an e-commerce social enterprise, Bricks & Order, and currently works in the UK as a freelance editor and researcher.

Alan Ducatman, MD, MS

Dr. Alan Ducatman is an internist and occupational physician. He is professor emeritus and former chair of the Department of Community Medicine and the interim founding dean of the School of Public Health at West Virginia University. His voluntary public service has included chairmanship of the US Accreditation Council on Graduate Medical Education's Residency Review Committee in Preventive Medicine, membership on the American Board of Preventive Medicine, and chairmanship of the external advising committee to the environmental health branches of the Centers for Disease Control and Prevention. Ducatman has devoted his clinical career to the prevention and mitigation of toxic exposures in workplaces and communities and has published extensively on the subject.

Ron Eller, PhD

Dr. Ron Eller is distinguished professor of history emeritus and former director of the Appalachian Center at the University of Kentucky. His published work includes *Miners, Millhands and Mountaineers: The Industrialization of the Appalachian South, 1880–1930* (1982) and *Uneven Ground: Appalachia since 1945* (2008 and 2012).

Angela Hagaman, DrPH(c), MA, NCC

Angela Hagaman serves as operations director of the East Tennessee State University Addiction Science Center. In this role she provides administrative and research support to faculty on a number of studies, including the National Institutes of Health–funded Studies to Advance Recovery Supports (STARS) in Central Appalachia and the HRSA-funded ETSU/NORC Rural Health Equity Research Center. She is also the principal investigator for the Tennessee Opioid SBIRT (Screening, Brief Intervention, and Referral to Treatment) project (TOS) with ETSU Family Medicine and coordinates several community-based prevention initiatives, including targeted outreach to the business community, active engagement with antidrug coalitions, and implementation of evidence-based curricula in schools and other youth-serving agencies. She has twelve years' experience working in the field of substance use prevention and treatment and is a national certified counselor. She is currently enrolled in ETSU's Doctor of Public Health Program.

Megan Heffernan, MPH

Megan Heffernan is a research scientist in NORC at the University of Chicago's Public Health Research Department. She is a seasoned rural health researcher, conducting projects related to substance use and public health systems and services. She has extensive expertise in qualitative and quantitative data collection and analysis and was instrumental in developing NORC's opioid misuse community assessment tool and Rural Prosperity Index. She currently serves on the editorial board of the *Journal of Public Health Management and Practice.*

Rachel Hogg-Graham, DrPH, MA

Dr. Rachel Hogg-Graham is an assistant professor in the Department of Health Management and Policy at the University of Kentucky College of Public Health. Her research focuses on cross-sector collaboration and the integration of health and social services.

Richard C. Ingram, DrPH, MEd

Dr. Richard Ingram is an associate professor at the University of Kentucky College of Public Health. His research interests include the oral health delivery system in the United States, the influence of variation in multisectoral collaboration on the delivery of population-based preventive services, and the impact of quality improvement initiatives, such as accreditation, on communities and the public health system.

Julie Marshall, PhD

Dr. Julie Marshall is an assistant professor at the Medical University of South Carolina (MUSC), with joint appointments in the James B. Edwards College of Dental Medicine's Division of Population Oral Health and the College of Medicine's Department of Public Health Sciences. Prior to joining MUSC, she was a senior economist at the Appalachian Regional Commission in Washington, DC, and served as Co-Principal Investigator on the Robert Wood Johnson Foundation's initiative Creating a Culture of Health in Appalachia. She was previously an economist for the US Congress's Joint Committee on Taxation, where her work contributed to creation of the 2010 Patient Protection and Affordable Care Act. Marshall's current research concentrates on rural health care, safety-net populations, social determinants of health and health disparities, and costs related to Medicaid-provided oral health care.

Stephanie M. Mathis, DrPH, MPH

Dr. Stephanie Mathis is an assistant professor of community and behavioral health, with an appointment to East Tennessee State University's Addiction Science Center (ASC). Her research interests include the prevention and treatment of prescription and other drug misuse, with an emphasis on intersections involving the fields of health communication and implementation science. In addition to providing leadership and support for ASC research activities, she provides evaluation support for community-based initiatives aligned with ASC.

Michael Meit, MA, MPH

Michael Meit serves as director of research and programs for the East Tennessee State University Center for Rural Health Research and as a senior fellow in NORC at the University of Chicago's Public Health Research Department. He recently led an Appalachian Regional Commission study of diseases of despair in Appalachia, which included the development of a companion Appalachian overdose mapping tool and the national expansion of that tool, the opioid misuse community assessment tool. Meit has experience working at both the state and national levels, including with the Pennsylvania Department of Health and the National Association of County and City Health Officials. He served as founding director of the University of Pittsburgh Center for Rural Health Practice, as codirector of NORC's Walsh Center for Rural Health Analysis, and on the boards of directors of the National Rural Health Association, Pennsylvania Public Health Association, and Maryland Rural Health Association. He currently serves on the American Public Health Association's Committee for Health Equity and on the editorial and advisory boards of the *Journal of Public Health Management and Practice, Journal of Appalachian Health*, and *Public Health Reports.*

Kelly E. Moore, PhD

Dr. Kelly E. Moore is a licensed clinical psychologist and assistant professor in the Department of Psychology at East Tennessee State University. She completed a postdoctoral fellowship in substance use prevention research at Yale School of Medicine. Her research interests include factors that contribute to poor adjustment after release from incarceration and the adaptation of evidence-based treatments for populations involved with the justice system. Much of Moore's work is related to understanding the psychological and behavioral consequences of the stigma associated with a criminal record.

Robert Pack, PhD, MPH

Dr. Robert Pack is a professor of community and behavioral health and associate dean for academic affairs at East Tennessee State University's College of Public Health. He is also director of the ETSU Addiction Science Center, the ETSU/NORC Rural Health Equity Research Center, and codirector of the Opioids Research Consortium of Central Appalachia. In 2018 the ETSU Addiction

Science Center won the US Public Health Service Award for Excellence in Interprofessional Education Collaboration. In 2019 Pack served on the Appalachian Regional Commission's Substance Abuse Advisory Council, on an expert panel for the Office of National Drug Control Policy, and as chair of the Association of Schools and Programs in Public Health Task Force on Public Health Approaches to Control the Epidemic of Opioid Use Disorder.

Margaret A. Riggs, PhD, MPH, MS

Dr. Margaret Riggs is a captain in the US Public Health Service and a senior epidemiologist at the Centers for Disease Control and Prevention (CDC). She serves as the healthy communities director for Shaping Our Appalachian Region, where she provides leadership and technical assistance to improve health in Appalachia Kentucky. She began her career as a CDC Epidemic Intelligence Service officer and has worked for the CDC since 2005 in the field of domestic and international public health, building public health preparedness and outbreak-response capacity. Riggs helped establish the Zambia National Public Health Institute and deployed for several large public health response efforts, including the COVID-19 pandemic, the Ebola virus outbreak in West Africa, Superstorm Sandy in New Jersey, the Haiti earthquake, tornadoes and an ice storm in Kentucky, and Hurricane Katrina in New Orleans.

James Alan Riley, PhD, MA

Dr. James Alan Riley has taught English and upper-level writing courses since 1987 at the University of Pikeville in Kentucky, where he currently serves as the undergraduate faculty chair. He is the recipient of a National Endowment for the Arts fellowship, two Al Smith fellowships from the Kentucky Arts Council, and an Individual Artists fellowship from the Ohio Arts Council. His most recent book is *Broken Frequencies: A Book of Poems* (2019), and he edited *Kentucky Voices: A Collection of Contemporary Kentucky Short Stories* (1997). His work has appeared in the *Journal of Kentucky Studies, Appalachian Heritage, Kentucky Monthly, Louisville Review, Kentucky Review, Connecticut Review, Greensboro Review*, and a variety of other journals and literary magazines. He served as the communications director for the Pike County government for a number of years under Judge Executive William "Bill" Deskins.

Ron R. Roach, PhD

Dr. Ron Roach is a professor and chair of the Department of Appalachian Studies and director of the Center of Excellence for Appalachian Studies and

Services at East Tennessee State University. He previously spent twelve years at Young Harris College in the north Georgia mountains, where he was the Maxwell professor of speech and the vice president for academic affairs; he also founded the college's Center for Appalachian Studies and Community Engagement. Roach has written about bluegrass festivals and the rhetoric of Appalachia, and has explored heritage tourism and comparative mountain studies in Scotland, Ireland, and the Carpathian Mountains of Ukraine and Romania. He directs the Appalachian Teaching Project for the ARC.

F. Douglas Scutchfield, MD

Dr. F. Douglas Scutchfield is a faculty fellow at the Lewis Honors College and the Peter P. Bosomworth Professor Emeritus in the College of Medicine and the College of Public Health, all at the University of Kentucky. He was responsible for creating the university's School of Public Health—now the College of Public Health. He was one of the founding faculty at the College of Community Health Sciences, as well as chair of the Department of Family and Community Medicine and associate dean, at the University of Alabama. Scutchfield also founded the Graduate School of Public Health at San Diego State University, where he is professor emeritus. He is the founder and the current editor in chief of the *Journal of Appalachian Health*. He has edited several books and has published extensively in the field of health.

Lindsay R. Stradtman, MPH, CPH

Lindsay Stradtman is a research program manager in the Department of Health, Behavior, and Society at the University of Kentucky College of Public Health. She has also worked with the university's Appalachian Center for Cancer Education, Screening, and Support and its Rural Cancer Prevention Center. She was previously a public health fellow at the Centers for Disease Control and Prevention. Her research efforts have involved health disparities in rural Appalachia, cancer prevention and control, and academic-community partnerships.

Erin Tanenbaum, MA

Erin Tanenbaum is a senior statistician at NORS at the University of Chicago. She has led dozens of analyses, from small rural health studies to large cross-functional studies, and is focused on improving health through predictive analytics and impact evaluation research. Tanenbaum is nationally recognized within the American Statistical Association (ASA), which has more than 19,000 members. She served as the elected chair of the ASA's Quality and Productivity

Chapter, was elected member at large of the Washington Statistical Society, was appointed chair of the Committee on Applied Statistics, and cofounded the ASA's mentoring program.

Logan Thomas, MA

Logan Thomas is an economist with the Appalachian Regional Commission. Since joining the ARC in May 2016, he has taken part in a number of research projects examining socioeconomic issues in the Appalachian region, including Creating a Culture of Health in Appalachia: Disparities and Bright Spots. Previously, he was part of a research team in the Division of Consumer and Community Affairs at the Federal Reserve Board of Governors, and he worked in the Department of Community Development for the City of Frostburg, Maryland.

Robin C. Vanderpool, DrPH

Dr. Robin Vanderpool is chief of the Health Communication and Informatics Research Branch of the Division of Cancer Control and Population Sciences at the National Cancer Institute. Prior to her tenure at NCI, she was a professor at the University of Kentucky College of Public Health and associate director for community outreach and engagement at the university's Markey Cancer Center. She has published extensively on the topics of rural health and cancer prevention and control.

Melissa White, MPH, MS

Melissa White is a doctoral student in the Department of Biostatistics and Epidemiology at East Tennessee State University's College of Public Health and a graduate assistant at the Center for Rural Health Research. Her research interests include chronic disease and nutritional epidemiology, as well as intergenerational cycles of poverty and health. White has been involved in research on diabetes education programs, adverse childhood experiences related to HIV adherence and retention, the relationship between poverty and adverse health outcomes in Appalachia, and the social determinants of health in Appalachia. She is currently studying prenatal, perinatal, and postpartum health as it relates to long-term health outcomes in rural, underserved populations.

Timothy Williams, DrPH, MS

Dr. Timothy Williams is a policy analyst at the Hilltop Institute at the University of Maryland, Baltimore County. He was formerly a research assistant at the Rural and Underserved Health Research Center and worked for several years as a substance abuse and mental health therapist in North Carolina, primarily in outpatient settings serving patients from rural areas.

Randy Wykoff, MD, MPH & TM

Dr. Randy Wykoff is founding dean of the College of Public Health and director of the Center for Rural Health Research at East Tennessee State University. He is a board-certified physician in both pediatrics and preventive medicine, with additional certification in tropical medicine. He previously served as senior vice president for international operations at Project HOPE and as the deputy assistant secretary for health in the US Department of Health and Human Services, which included a year as the acting executive director of the President's Council on Physical Fitness and Sport. During eleven years at the Food and Drug Administration, he was associate commissioner for AIDS and special health issues, followed by a detail with Senator Edward Kennedy and the Senate Labor and Human Resources Committee and, later, a stint as associate commissioner for operations, which included eighteen months as deputy to the acting commissioner. Wykoff began his career as district medical director of the Upper Savannah Health District in the South Carolina Department of Health and Environmental Control.

Katherine Youngen, MPH

Katherine Youngen is a health policy researcher with a focus on health inequities and underserved populations. Her master of public health from the University of Kentucky College of Public Health includes a concentration in health policy.

Index

Understanding and Improving Health for Minority and Disadvantaged Populations

Series Editor: F. Douglas Scutchfield

This series investigates the nature and character of current public health and medical care issues for specific disadvantaged and minority populations in the United States. It also seeks to examine the medical care status and concerns that impact the care these populations receive. Books in this series suggest new approaches based on evidence-driven solutions to the inequities that members of these groups face in health. This series includes coverage of Appalachian, Black, Indigenous, Latinx, and refugee populations, among others, and examines challenges that disproportionately affect these groups. Books in this series describe the notion of socioecological determinants within these populations and examine efforts to mitigate for these determinants. The texts are intended for public health students, educators, and policymakers, as well as the educated lay person with an interest in public health topics and solutions for these marginalized populations.